PRAISE FOR *INCONCEIVABLE*

"This book will make any reader feel stronger, no matter what their medical politics."

—*Library Journal*

"A sensational book . . . honest and beautifully heartfelt."

—Dr. Wayne W. Dyer, bestselling author of
Your Erroneous Zones

"A terrific book that shows couples how to help themselves through positive lifestyle changes and mind-body work. A powerful complement to medical treatment."

—Marc Goldstein, M.D., F.A.C.S., Co-Executive Director,
Cornell Institute for Reproductive Medicine;
Professor of Reproductive Medicine,
Cornell University, Weil Medical College;
coauthor of *The Couple's Guide to Fertility*

"It's nice to read a medical story with a happy ending. It's even nicer when we learn something useful from it for our own lives. So it is with Julia Indichova's mindful journey described in *Inconceivable*."

—Ellen Langer, Ph.D., Professor of Psychology,
Harvard Medical School; author of *Mindfulness*

"When inspiration and information are combined there is no limit to what one may create. Read this and learn that what you can conceive of can be achieved."

—Bernie Siegel, M.D., bestselling author of
Love, Medicine and Miracles

"I would love all my patients to fight for themselves with the strength of Ms. Indichova's commitment. Her demanding self-analysis, good humor, and determination just fly off the page. It's magic."

—Alan Natow, M.D., Clinical Associate Professor,
New York University School of Medicine

"This is an empowering book—and a delightful read. We learn that strengthening one's body through natural means can reap lasting spiritual and physical benefits, and possibly tip the balance in favor of conception."

—Carolyn Berger, Chair, American Infertility Association

"Julia Indichova's book is remarkable in that it opens the reader's eyes to the possibility of turning the infertility struggle into a positive physical and emotional experience—one way or another."

—Jane T., Resolve of Northern California

"This revealing narrative shows that for some individuals a positive mind-set and alternative medicine may be as powerful as traditional fertility drugs."

—Sami David, M.D., gynecologist/fertility specialist

"This courageous and heartwarming story inspires us to look beyond statistics and shows that emotionally and physically based holistic therapies can encourage conception."

—Niravi B. Payne, M.S., author of
The Whole Person Fertility Program

"A treat and a delight! This is not a book about infertility. It is really about the process of inner growth, triggered by the circumstances of her (Indichova's) infertility; will benefit anyone interested in transforming their life."

—Aquarius, Atlanta

"Any book worth reading will give you a good read and the chance to connect with someone beyond your immediate circle. A very good book can very well change your life. *Inconceivable* is such a book."

—Lois Nachamie, author, *So Glad We Waited:*
A Hand-holding Guide
for Parents over 35

"A narrative filled with humor, heartache, and ultimately hope."

—*Healthy Living*

". . . Will inspire not only people seeking pregnancy, but anyone with long-term health problems who needs to learn to trust their own instincts."

—*Jewish Voice*

INCONCEIVABLE

A Woman's

Triumph over

Despair and

Statistics

INCONCEIVABLE

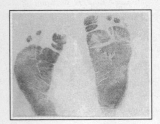

JULIA INDICHOVA

BROADWAY BOOKS   New York

BROADWAY

This book is not intended to take the place of medical advice from a trained medical professional. Readers are advised to consult a physician or other qualified health professional regarding treatment of their medical problems. Neither the publisher nor the author takes any responsibility for any possible consequences from any treatment, action, or application of medicine, herb, or preparation to any person reading or following the information in this book.

A hardcover edition of this book was originally self-published in 1997 by Adell Press. It is here reprinted by arrangement with Adell Press.

Broadway Books titles may be purchased for business or promotional use or for special sales. For information, please write to: Special Markets Department, Random House, Inc., 1540 Broadway, New York, NY 10036.

BROADWAY BOOKS and its logo, a letter B bisected on the diagonal, are trademarks of Broadway Books, a division of Random House, Inc.

Visit our website at www.broadwaybooks.com

First Broadway Books trade paperback edition published 2001

Designed by Helene Berinsky

Library of Congress Cataloging-in-Publication Data

Indichova, Julia.
    Inconceivable: a woman's triumph over despair and statistics / Julia Indichova.
        p.   cm.
    Includes bibliographical references.
        1. Indichova, Julia.   2. Infertility, Female—Patients—Biography.   I. Title.
    RG201 .I53 2001
362.1'98178'0092—dc21
[B]   2001035492

ISBN 0-7679-0820-1

10   9   8   7   6   5   4   3   2   1

In celebration of my parents

Edita Lenorovich

and Oskar Indich.

Their memory is for me a

source of countless blessings.

CONTENTS

Contents

FOREWORD

Ever since its publication in 1998, I've been recommending Julia Indichova's wonderful book, *Inconceivable,* not only to women seeking pregnancy, but to anyone interested in deciphering the messages behind symptoms. Julia's story is powerful medicine. It expands our concept of fertility far beyond eggs, sperm, and babies, allowing us to become fertile ground for new ideas and creations. The story also provides a stunning example of turning a health crisis into an opportunity for discovery, transformation, and growth.

Given the current scientific understanding of fertility, Julia's healthy pregnancy and birth shouldn't have happened. And they wouldn't have if she had simply gone along with what multiple doctors told her was true. Julia had the courage to do something else. She listened to her inner wisdom—that still, small voice within that comes to us in dreams, in hunches, in gut feelings. That inner voice *xiv* that tells us to have faith and believe despite all evidence to the contrary. As a result, Julia entered a whole new world. A world in which our physical bodies begin to respond more to what is possible than to statistical probabilities. By following her inner wisdom and by learning to care for her body on every level, Julia began to increase her life energy, her chi as it's called in Chinese medicine. She quite literally made herself a sound container for conceiving and nurturing new life. And this happened by first paying attention to and healing the only physical body and life force she had dominion over: her own. This is the heart of the matter. When we're willing to listen to our bodies and begin trusting ourselves as much as we trust outer authorities, all the rules change. And so does our biology. Statistics no longer apply to us. We enter the realm of miracles and undreamed-of possibilities. As soon as we open to what is possible, our bodies also begin to change.

When I think back on my ob/gyn training in the 1970s, I am struck by how different the world was then. In one of the Catholic hospitals where I did deliveries, scores of forty-somethings got pregnant all the time. The problem for these women, many of whom had four or more children at home, wasn't how to get pregnant. It was how to avoid pregnancy. Brant Secunda, a medicine man from the remote Mexican Huichol tribe, says that women in that tribe routinely get pregnant well beyond what our society considers "the childbearing years." They don't get cable TV or the Internet. No one has told them that their eggs are too old. They simply believe that the female body is a sacred vessel that can produce life. And, as a result, it is.

Each of us is part of the culture in which we were born and raised and we are influenced in body, mind, and spirit by that culture throughout our lives. At the same time, cultures change, evolve, and heal because of the courage of individuals. Julia Indichova is one of those individuals. Let her be an inspiration for you of how to trust yourself, heal yourself, and reconnect with the wonder of your body and all of its possibilities.

—Christiane Northrup, M.D., author of
Women's Bodies, Women's Wisdom

*If this life be not a real fight, in which something
is eternally gained for the universe by success,
it is no better than a game of private theatricals
from which one may withdraw at will.
But it feels like a real fight.*

—WILLIAM JAMES

Inconceivable

INTRODUCTION

Although I had never aspired to become an author, the writing of this book became somewhat of an obsession. A sense of gratitude, obligation, and urgency drew me toward my computer: gratitude for my two glorious children, obligation to share what I learned with others, and urgency to send this story on its way, knowing someone out there is waiting to hear it.

Several years ago I was that someone. At the age of forty-two, only thirteen months after the birth of my first child, my FSH (follicle-stimulating hormone) level was the same as my age, 42. According to specialists in reproductive medicine, it was a clear indication that my body was no longer producing fertilizable eggs.

After the diagnosis, I searched in vain for information that presented an alternative to their recommendations. It would have meant a great deal to me to learn about others

2 who had won the fertility battle despite the medical establishment's prognosis.

Shortly after the birth of my second child, friends started circulating the story of my "miraculous" pregnancy. My husband became the much sought-after fertility adviser among his colleagues at Bear Stearns, where he worked as a computer programmer. He often came home with stories of miscarriages, multiple in vitro fertilization trials, and unexplained infertility. Though I never met most of the people he talked about, I felt a strong connection with them. In my mind's eye I saw them rummaging through "how to get pregnant" books at the local bookstore, giving their names to the receptionist of the latest fertility guru, listening to the recorded message of the IVF clinic of their choice. I heard their disillusioned sighs as they saw another month go by without the promise of parenthood.

What if reading my story could make them take a step back? It might be just enough to stop all the voices pointing them in a hundred directions. Just enough to realize that the answers they come up with on their own could be as significant as the answers of the experts, that no one else's motivation to give them what they want can be as powerful as their own, no one's resolve stronger, no one's intuition keener; that not a single specialist is as close to their own bodies and souls as they are. Perhaps reading my story could encourage others diagnosed with fertility problems as well as other chronic ailments to do something out of character: go to a yoga class, try a glass of fresh vegetable juice, or learn about Eastern medicine.

Certainly, no one can guarantee that our efforts will   *3*
crack the code and bring us the result we hope for. The
only thing that is certain is that taking an active part in the
treatment process leaves less room for despair. It creates op-
portunities we could not have anticipated. In the last seven
years of working with people in my workshops, support
groups, and through my website FertileHeart.com, it has
become clear to me that sewn deep in the lining of the most
unattractive garment—whether it's labeled infertility, fi-
bromyalgia, depression, or any other name—is a precious
gem. Our task is to find that gem; discover what it is for
each of us and to draw strength from the search.

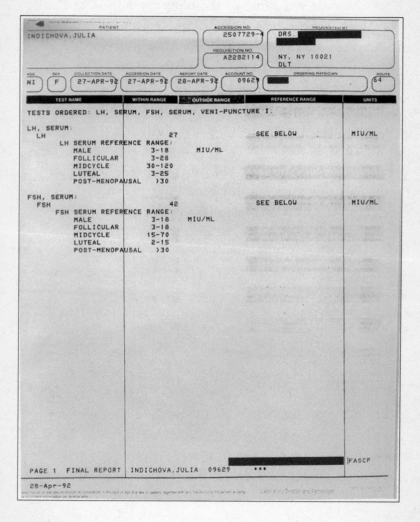

INDICHOVA, JULIA | 2507729-4 | DRS.

REQUISITION NO. | A2282114 | NY, NY 10021 DLT

AGE	SEX	COLLECTION DATE	ACCESSION DATE	REPORT DATE	ACCOUNT NO.	ORDERING PHYSICIAN	ROUTE
NI	F	27-APR-92	27-APR-92	28-APR-92	09629		64

TEST NAME	WITHIN RANGE	OUTSIDE RANGE	REFERENCE RANGE	UNITS

TESTS ORDERED: LH, SERUM, FSH, SERUM, VENI-PUNCTURE I.

LH, SERUM:
```
  LH                          27                    SEE BELOW        MIU/ML
          LH SERUM REFERENCE RANGE:
                  MALE          3-18      MIU/ML
                  FOLLICULAR    3-28
                  MIDCYCLE      30-120
                  LUTEAL        3-25
                  POST-MENOPAUSAL  >30

FSH, SERUM:
  FSH                         42                    SEE BELOW        MIU/ML
          FSH SERUM REFERENCE RANGE:
                  MALE          3-18      MIU/ML
                  FOLLICULAR    3-18
                  MIDCYCLE      15-70
                  LUTEAL        2-15
                  POST-MENOPAUSAL  >30
```

FASCP

PAGE 1   FINAL REPORT   INDICHOVA, JULIA   09629   * * *

28-Apr-92

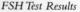

FSH Test Results

1

DIAGNOSIS

Oh, if there were in me one seed without rust . . .

—CZESLAW MILOSZ, *The Song*

I love teaching. After twenty years of working in the theater, I recently got a master's degree and was lucky enough to land a job teaching Russian and musical comedy in the hottest junior high school in Manhattan.

But Kathryn, our daughter's baby-sitter, has quit. Now Ellena wants to have nothing to do with any of the possible replacements. Except one. Me. She is only ten months old, and every time I leave the room her wailing reels me back in. There is only one thing to do: stay home until she becomes more comfortable with new people.

After a couple of weeks at home, I realize Kathryn's sudden departure was a gift. I would never have dared to choose full-time motherhood over work. Never found out how much I enjoyed the preciously unhurried hours with my daughter: cruising with the baby backpack through our morning errands, walking around the Columbia University campus just north of us, or savoring our raisin bagel in the nearby bakery. We live in a fifteen-story prewar building across from Riverside Park, and if I lean far enough out the kitchen window, I can see a patch of green. It's not unusual to meet up with a cluster of park-bound strollers in the lobby. Within a week, Ellena and I are part of a neighbor-hood play group. As long as we can manage financially, I will teach in the evenings and continue being a full-time mom. Thankfully, my husband, Ed, supports my decision.

There is an added bonus to all this. With no teaching schedule to consider, the second baby could come anytime. Let's see, if it arrived nine months from now, my two chil-dren would be only nineteen months apart. Lying in bed at night, I take a deep breath and imagine movement under the slope of my belly. I see myself lean against the weight of a double stroller and wonder whether it will fit through our front door.

Three months later, I'm still a full-time mom, now a part-time teacher of English to speakers of other languages at Hunter College. It seems Ellena's sibling is taking a little longer than we anticipated. I'm not really concerned. After all, the last time I got pregnant on the first try. Three months is not very long. But I'm forty-two. A consultation with my gynecologist might be in order.

"We should take an FSH test," suggests Dr. Y. "It's one of the first things we look at in women over forty." A week later I call for the results.

"Oh, yes," reports the nurse, "your numbers are fine,

within normal range." A sigh of relief, a phone call to Ed, all is well. In a few days I call to schedule further testing. I am stunned to find out that, although the numbers are not "abnormal," all is not well.

"The follicle-stimulating hormone helps the follicles inside your ovaries to develop into eggs. If the level is—over 20—" Dr. Y pauses—"your ovaries are not working as well as they should be. With an FSH of 42 there is not much I can do for you. You'll need to see a fertility specialist."

I sleepwalk through the rest of the day. How could I have been so arrogant, ignoring my age? Did I think my biological clock had stopped ticking just because it took me so long to find the right man? We should have started trying sooner. And what is my problem? Why does this hurt so much when I already have the most wonderful daughter in the world? How dare I lament with all those childless couples out there? Yet I can't undo the feeling of despair. I know how much Ed wants to have another child and how much we would love Ellena to have a sibling. Dr. Y refers me to a specialist. That must mean a specialist can help.

Dr. N strikes the first blow.

"I'm sorry," says the receptionist. "Dr. N will not accept you as a patient. Your FSH is too high. He doesn't feel he could help you." A decent man, he is saving me money. Yet all I hear is that it's so bad, he doesn't even want to try.

"What happened? You look sick," says Ed as soon as he opens the door. Of course, he's shocked. Last week there was nothing in our way except a few months of practice until we got it right. My impulse for self-flagellation wins out once again: "If only we had started right after Ellena's birth. They say that's the most fertile time. We should've known!"

A line of fear cuts across his face, but he is enlightened, as always: "We couldn't have moved any faster, we were not ready. Everything will work out. Do you remember when we first held Ellena? How tiny she was? How easy it was to love her? We'll love this baby no matter where it comes from."

Ed is right. I mustn't for a moment forget how lucky I am. Ellena, Ellenka. Her name combines the names of her two grandmothers (Edita, Helen) for double protection. In return she carries sparks of them in her blue eyes, the color and texture of her sun-bathed hair. I must be there for her. I can't give in to the feeling of defeat that sneaks up on me when I least expect it.

My friend Lisa and I went to college together. Our relationship has gone through its ups and downs, but still my hand automatically dials her number in times of crisis. She and her husband, Gary, have been members of the infertility subculture for the past four years, having gone from specialist to specialist to finally adopting their son, Sam, three months ago.

"This is the worst part, when they tell you something's wrong. It gets easier after that," says Lisa.

On Lisa's recommendation I call Resolve, a national organization for people with infertility problems. They might have some new information. I'm hoping for a recent breakthrough in research, someone to discount the FSH alarmists.

I leave a message briefly describing my situation. The woman who returns my call, Shelly, is only thirty-seven. She has an FSH problem as well. Like me, she has one biological child, though she had trouble conceiving the first time. Our hormone levels create an instant bond.

"I know how you feel," Shelly says sympathetically. "Our doctor suggested IVF, but it's not an option for us. We can't go through it again. We're in the midst of the adoption process."

I ask her if she ever tried alternative treatments. "Like herbs? No, not really," she replies. "I guess you never know, do you?"

Across a haze of information, a list of doctors and IVF clinics, I hear a certain resignation, a weariness I fear might be contagious.

The complimentary Resolve newsletter arrives a few days later with an entire page filled with information on support groups. I am not ready to join one, but it's comforting to know they're there.

I'm surprised no one mentioned the effect of a high FSH on your environment. Seemingly overnight the entire Upper West Side of Manhattan swells into a giant, mocking belly. The playgrounds are invaded with mothers expecting their second or third child, or cradling newborns against their breasts. It seems almost daily there is joyous news of yet another one of Ellena's playmates becoming a big brother or sister. Each time the news feels like a humiliating betrayal to me.

Dr. C is at the top of Lisa's list of referrals. Getting an

appointment is surprisingly easy. His office is on the street level of a lovely brownstone in Greenwich Village. Ed takes a late lunch hour to meet me for a two-thirty appointment. Finally, my first specialist.

A young woman with two screeching bundles is holding court in his waiting room. That's what I call a good omen. "They're Pergonal babies," she says to no one in particular. "We worked hard for them."

I imagine her gravely injecting her thigh while staring at a Gerber baby taped on her refrigerator door for inspiration. She walks out energized by her new motherhood and proceeds to load her car with the precious cargo.

Dr. C is an elegant, gray-haired man in his late fifties. On his desk sits a photograph of a beautiful woman holding twin girls. His daughters? Maybe his very first Pergonal twins? Nothing's sacred anymore.

Unaware of my silent indiscretion, Dr. C begins to take a brief medical history. He asks me about first menstruation, first pregnancy, Ellena's birth, and the regularity and duration of my ovulation cycles, all of which he finds satisfactory. Prior to this visit, Ed was asked to get a sperm count, and it's comforting to know we're not lacking in that department.

Dr. C looks at the lab report with my FSH. "Forty-two is high. Very high," he says, sounding concerned.

"Doesn't the number fluctuate? Couldn't it just drop on its own?"

"Of course it could, but the fact that it even once went up this high is discouraging. Ordinarily, I would recommend Pergonal. It's a fertility drug that helps you release more mature eggs. You could administer it to yourself by daily injections into your buttocks. Only, I don't think with these numbers it would do much good. I wouldn't want to give you any false hope. The prognosis is poor. In vitro fertilization is an option. Of course, you would have to get an egg donor.

"I still think we should run all the basic tests," he adds. "To make sure everything else is all right. And you'll need to have them if you elect to go the IVF route. One more thing: before we schedule the tests I'd like you to meet with our staff psychologist, Dr. R.

"Hope we can help," he says, shaking hands. Later I hear him repeat the phrase to another desperate, smiling couple.

Three weeks later, as we go through subsequent visits and discuss lab results and additional options over the phone, it becomes quite clear Dr. C has no idea who I am. Literally. I have a feeling he loses track of his patients in the maze of sonograms, biopsies, sperm counts, and referrals. Maybe he doesn't need to know me, as long as he knows his trade. As long as he updates my chart. Knows not to give me too much or too little of anything. Knows how to take a snip off my uterine wall and not hurt me more than he has to. So what if he thinks I'm the tall blonde instead of the short brunette?

The next step is our appointment with Dr. R, the psychologist.

She greets us in the waiting room. "Don't worry, I have

everything under control," says her neatly tailored dark suit and her breezy smile. For a moment I'm reminded of those flawless faces one sees behind the make-up counters at Bloomingdale's. A dab of color, a stroke of a brush and you're as good as new. Instead of glamorous photographs, the walls of her office are covered with colorful diagrams of the female reproductive system; on her desk lies a plastic model of a uterus and ovaries, and a couple of syringes.

The first order of business is to reassure me I'm not going through menopause. "Women seem to think a high FSH means menopause is just around the corner," she says, "but of course it doesn't mean that at all." She is pleased to be the bearer of such good news, happy to clear up a foolish yet understandable error.

"Does that mean I can have another baby?" I ask.

"Unfortunately," she continues, "it does mean your ovaries are no longer producing fertilizable eggs. Now there are a number of procedures to compensate for this, various fertility drugs to boost the production of eggs and to improve their quality. In your case, however, the FSH is too high to merit the use of any of them. The only thing Dr. C recommends is IVF with an egg donor or, if you want guaranteed results, adoption, or surrogacy." She hands Ed a business card of a therapist specializing in adoption, and another of a lawyer who helps couples find surrogates.

Before we leave, Dr. R gives us a description of ovaries enlarged by doses of Pergonal. If I elect to do IVF, taking Pergonal is part of the process. "You would be closely monitored, but it's a powerful drug.

"And no," she says in response to Ed's last question, "there is no documented case of anyone conceiving with these numbers."

A quiet moaning starts up at the base of my abdomen, and I reach for Ed's hand. His fingers wrap around my palm. I need to get out of here, but it seems Dr. R is waiting for some sort of, preferably emotional, response from the two of us. Something to justify our presence in her office. Otherwise why would a consultation with her be part of the routine? A prerequisite for the rest of the tests? To provide us with a professional shoulder to cry on? In case, after fifteen years of analysis, I might not be aware of needing a therapist? Or was it to hear Dr. C's diagnosis produced by a different set of vocal cords? Or could it be that this conference was dictated largely by the rising cost of commercial real estate?

One thing is clear: the fertility roller coaster is in motion. And like it or not, I'm on it.

2

Off to See the Wizards

"She told my uterus to stop bleeding and it did. And then she spoke to the sac in a quiet, gentle voice. The way one would talk to a small child: 'Okay, you bled enough, now you can stop.' And the blood stopped. Then she showed Allen how to cut the umbilical cord with dental floss."

I'm listening to a testimonial to the otherworldly powers of Karen's midwife, Joanne. She helped Karen deliver her baby in a home birth without any accoutrements of modern medicine.

"She seemed to have absolute faith in what she was doing. It was contagious. It made me trust her," Karen says, absentmindedly digging a small green toy shovel into the sand.

You can't get any more New Age or spiritual than Karen:

teaching an herb class in the East Village, driving sixty miles to bury her placenta under a mulberry tree that fed her berries the previous summer, hard at work on a novel about an eleven-year-old mystic who lives in a hole. Karen is someone who'll stop in the middle of the street and say, "Oh, no wonder all men look so good today, it's almost a full moon." Karen is in touch. I trust her intuition about people. Besides, if Karen's uterus responded so readily to Joanne, maybe my ovaries will do the same. Maybe Joanne could have a little chat with them. Maybe she knows some secret code. It's not that strange. People talk to plants.

"You could just call her," says Karen. "See what she has to say. She might recommend someone."

"What's there to lose?" we intone in unison.

Joanne sounds very matter-of-fact about being able to help me: "I work with a Native American medicine man and we've had a hundred percent success rate." She needs to check on the healer's availability. My appointment is confirmed the next day. Boy, a hundred percent success rate sounds good.

Just the act of scheduling an appointment feels like the Red Cross just landed with fresh supplies. The possibility of new answers makes the diagnosis less final, less devastating. There are people out there who are not writing me off, healers in their own right, even if they're not licensed physicians. I told her my age, I told her the diagnosis, and she didn't hang up on me. That's something.

For the next week, I entertain colorful visions of

16   shamans engaged in ritual dance. They search the sky for
omens, then lift my body high above their heads and chant
in a strange language.

A Native American medicine man. Sounds promising. I
imagine the finely chiseled face of a mystic bending over me.
Deliberate in his movements, he transforms himself into a
living channel between me and the healing forces of nature.

I flash to a documentary on the rain forests in which the
guide pointed to a plant, saying: "When a woman decides
she no longer wants to bear children, she eats a mouthful of
these."

I bet he'll have a number of useful tips. There must be
so much I can learn from him. He'll cajole the spirits of
procreation to rush to my rescue.

The healer and the midwife both live and practice in
New Jersey, not the most geographically desirable location.
The mere mention of New Jersey sends a flare of panic
through my nervous system. It jolts me back to my first
taste of America in 1969: my elderly uncle's childless home
on the corner of a dead-end street in Fair Lawn. The street
was lined with identical houses whose occupants came and
went without ever being seen. Not a single soul could be
spied through the curtained windows.

Having just completed my first year at the University of
Performing Arts in Bratislava, I intended to go back and
continue my studies in September. But everyone urged me
to stay. Aunt Lilli spent hours helping me with my English;
uncle Nick wrote letters to politicians to help secure my
immigrant status.

I might as well have landed on Mars. The middle-class New Jersey suburb I found myself in was unlike anything I had ever experienced. My uncle's friends and their children were assigned the tedious task of entertaining Nick's "nice young niece." Her parents, they were told, were part of a small Hungarian Jewish community in Czechoslovakia and the poor girl escaped the tentacles of Communism by the skin of her teeth.

"What a drag," I could hear them thinking as they politely opened the door on the passenger side of their father's Oldsmobile. "She doesn't speak a word of English; she looks totally shell-shocked; and she sure as hell isn't gonna put out."

New Jersey meant being an ill-formed alien as I tried to wrap my tongue around the cumbersome sounds of a new language. New Jersey was being a foreigner.

But today New Jersey is where I go to be healed.

Boarding the bus at Port Authority and settling into the red vinyl seats of the Red and Tan line, I remind myself of the reason for this venture. William, the healer, comes well recommended. If Karen thinks I should see him, that's reason enough to do it. He might hold the missing piece of the puzzle, something small but significant. As long as there's a possibility of learning something new, I can't afford not to follow through.

I get off the bus in the middle of a small suburb, clutching my notebook with the directions. Turn right, look for Maple Avenue. The street is typically deserted. I keep walking in spite of what's become an involuntary mantra in my head: "What am I doing here?"

"Resistance, resistance," chimes my overanalyzed psyche.

My fears will dissolve as soon as I meet Joanne and William, I say to myself. It's just this lack of human form that makes me a little anxious. I'm walking through a perfectly ordinary middle-class neighborhood to meet an American Indian medicine man. What's so strange about that? Who said enlightenment can't dwell behind a white screen door?

"You're looking for William?" asks a lanky young man, about eighteen, standing behind the door, before my hand reaches the doorbell. "He'll be with you in a few minutes. Have a seat." Off he goes to rejoin the basketball game in the backyard. Ten minutes pass, and I'm beginning to feel mildly irritated.

In a little while Joanne enters, blue-eyed and windburned, with a pitcher of pungent raspberry tea. "William is with another client at the moment," she says as she ushers me to what appears to be the room of her teenage daughter. After several minutes of polite exchanges unrelated to the nature of my visit, she instructs me to meditate. "It's a good way to open yourself up to the healing process," she says reassuringly. Wait a minute, I didn't come here to meditate. C'mon, lady, I have a million questions, I think. She walks briskly out of the room before the words can roll off my tongue.

I close my eyes and focus on my breath, trying to screen out the basketball being dribbled, its repeated thump against the metal ridge of the hoop. What am I doing? I should be meditating. My lack of concentration might be the very thing that will hinder the effectiveness of the treatment.

Still, the room with all its teenage paraphernalia demands my attention. Collections of dolls, glass bowls filled with pastel-colored crystals. A vanity strewn with hair ornaments, earrings. A small bunch of dried flowers in a miniature hand-painted vase. A white jean jacket draped over a chair. What if it gets chilly and she needs her jacket? What if she bursts into the room, finds me gaping at her possessions, and screams, "Mom, what is she doing in here? You're always having strangers in my room," her face flushed with indignant adolescent rage?

But no one comes. I've been here almost an hour. Is this what I'm paying a hundred and fifty dollars for? I wrestle with the impulse to leave, to tell the midwife that this is beginning to feel like a rip-off. Or I could just make something up.

What am I afraid of? Do I think she will chase me down the street with a broom shouting obscenities? No, it's not the midwife I'm afraid of. I'm afraid that I might miss something. That this may be an opportunity unrecognized by me. That there is something here that could be IT. It's just my resistance, I tell myself, willing my mind to settle down and focus. I'm sure they have this all mapped out; they know what works.

As if to reward me for my renewed faith, Joanne comes to escort me to the master bedroom on the top floor. "William has just ended a very strenuous session. He needs a few minutes to refuel," she says. Once again, she tells me

20   to sit on the bed and continue my meditation. I guess the air in the bedroom, dense with procreation, is supposed to work its magic on me.

Resistance or not, I have a distinct feeling that something is off. They are trying to make it look like this is all part of the routine, when in fact they're just stalling for time. Has there been a scheduling error? I can't believe this is the standard sequence of events. Maybe there's a back door. It's not too late. I could sneak out. But of course, I stay. William should be here any minute.

And there he is. At last. First there is a sound of heaving, followed by a brief rhythmic huffing and puffing. Enter William. He is a large, middle-aged man, a taut belly ballooning over his belt. He could easily be cast as the neighbor who stops by for a bit of football watching and beer.

Settle down, Julia, I chide myself, he is not here to audition for a Kevin Costner movie. He is here to bestow on you the age-old wisdom of people who know how to tap into the healing powers of Mother Nature.

"So how can I help you?" he asks jovially. "Oh well. Your husband is going to have to help you with that. By the way, are you having intercourse?"

"Sometimes as much as three times a day," I tell him, trying to match his whimsical tone.

I proceed to tell him about my FSH problem and the poor prognosis. He nods and says cheerfully, "Oh, you're lucky. You've only been trying a few months. Some of these people that come to see me have been at it for years.

One couple came to me after ten years. I advised them to adopt and wouldn't you know it, she got pregnant a few months after the arrival of their son. Happens a lot. You're lucky. You probably just need a minor adjustment."

I wonder what he'd say if I just got up and left, I think, lying on Joanne's king-size marriage bed. William starts to press down on my chest bones. "By massaging the chest bones in an upward direction you're giving your organs more space, more breathing room. You need to do this twice a day, each time for about fifteen minutes. I wouldn't worry. Your problem is insignificant. Be sure to keep the channel of communication between you and your husband free of interference. When is the next bus to the city?"

He walks me downstairs, suddenly anxious to put me on the bus and once again in urgent need of sustenance. He seems annoyed at Joanne, who responds with an air of someone who has been repeatedly chastised for a recurring error. Is it always like this? Or did something go wrong today?

Joanne offers to drive me to the bus station. She is an herbalist in addition to being a midwife, and I was to get a list of herbs from her. "We can do a quick herbal consultation if we have time. If not, we'll do it over the phone," she says, putting the key into the ignition.

At the bus stop, standing in the least conspicuous spot behind a phone booth, we face each other. Joanne instructs me to raise both arms parallel to the ground. "Now we will ask your body which herbs would be most appropriate for you," she says, going through a list of herbs and intermit-

22   tently pressing down on my outstretched arms. If my arms resist the pressure, the herb is not for me.

The bus is here. I hand her my check for a hundred and fifty dollars. A few minutes later I'm on my way home, numb with rage and disappointment.

After a few days my anger subsides and the episode takes on the flavor of a New Age sitcom, especially after Karen's husband, Allen, gives me his own take on the enterprising little sales team.

"I'm not at all surprised this didn't work for you," he says, sitting on the stool in our kitchen. He tugs at his beard and chuckles. "I must say Joanne was suspect from the beginning. She told us she attended a hundred births, which is a mysteriously round number. Don't you think?"

"I do think," I say, remembering the hundred percent success rate.

"It's true, she was very good for us," Allen continues, getting a bottle of apple juice from the refrigerator, "but it was mainly because Karen had great faith in her. You see, she saw Joanne as a saintly figure. Kind of the way Joanne sees herself. Karen had implicit faith in her and Joanne had implicit faith in herself, so between the two of them they had a good birth. Karen accepted everything. Even the idea of putting Krazy Glue on a herpes sore in case she had a breakout. Joanne presented it as the most irrefutable procedure and we went along." He grins at me, sipping his juice. "She also told Karen it was within her power to choose not to have a breakout at the time of the birth and luckily, she didn't.

"Oh yeah, William." He laughs when I mention Joanne's partner. "It seems to me he's a suburban guru with a tenuous Native American connection, who has a number of followers and who exploits the fact that American Indians are very chic nowadays. Karen went to a number of his talks and she always came back with a headache, kicking herself for not being able to understand this man's wisdom.

"Karen would not agree with me," continues Allen, "but I kind of see him and Joanne as a couple of con artists working in the American tradition of selling faith. If you sell faith it sometimes succeeds. Karen was capable of believing in this person, you weren't. Also, I think your problem is a little more complex. We just needed a midwife." *Ai, yai, yai,* the Hungarian *woe is me,* I moan silently. Allen is right. I guess my faith didn't stretch all the way to New Jersey.

Later I learn that other, solid midwives know a great deal about pregnancy and birth. But for the time being, I'm staying in New York, with certified fertility specialists, as mainstream as they come in their nondeviant Park Avenue offices.

3

OFF AND RUNNING

With all the talk about the rapid decline of reproductive organs after a certain age and the reminders of time as the great enemy, I wouldn't be surprised to find an oversized hourglass on the desk of the next specialist. Its hypersensitive mechanism would give an instant reading of one's ovaries and automatically siphon off the appropriate volume of sand. In my case, it says, the sand has already run out.

Still, in spite of what they tell me, I have a feeling that if I run fast enough I can still make it. I come across a line in a Czeslaw Milosz poem: *"Oh, if there were in me one seed without rust . . ."* I must find a doctor who will be willing to work with me, someone to help me unearth that one untarnished seed.

Ed's cousin, Annie, a dermatologist, suggests I get tested again to see if there is any change. This time my FSH is 34, an eight-point drop from the original number. Perhaps now I qualify to become Dr. N's patient. If he accepts me, that means I am salvageable. I ask Lisa to make the call in case the nurse recognizes my accent and remembers I'd already been shooed away before. Once again, we need to wait until the nurse calls back with Dr. N's response.

"It's still too high," says Lisa, then adds, "Welcome to the world of fertility doctors." Was there a trace of sarcasm in her tone?

Am I imagining the discomfort of some of the pregnant women I know from the park? Walking into the bagel store today, I see Jane, one of the playground moms I used to spend time with last summer. I haven't seen her for a while. Her coat is open. Looking at her swollen belly, I suddenly remember sitting around the baby slide with her and two other women, telling them Ed and I were going to start working on the second baby. Jane looked at me then and groaned, "I definitely need a little break."

Two years later, here she is and here I am. She seemed uncomfortable seeing me. She remembered our conversation. She knows. Everyone knows.

I may be getting a little paranoid. Going to one Resolve meeting doesn't necessarily mean I'll walk out with a scarlet "I" burned into my forehead. It might help me feel less isolated.

The woman I spoke to on the Resolve hot line mentioned an informal drop-in support group, which meets each month. On the way to the meeting I envision an auditorium filled with small clusters of women and men with

26   their heads together, reviewing strategies. I hear the echoes
of the countless marches of my girlhood as a Communist
fledgling: "Those who don't join our march are against us,
but they will not sway us from our path."

I am fifteen minutes late. A dozen or so women and a
few men sit around a large oval conference table. A young
woman with long dark hair who looks to be in her late
twenties has the floor: "The waiting stage is the hardest for
me. The two weeks of waiting to find out if it worked." A
woman's voice breaks in from the far end of the table: "Oh,
it's agonizing. Every time I feel a cramp I want to call my
doctor and ask, can I still be pregnant if I feel a cramp."

A tall woman in her forties is looking for a referral: "The
clinic we're working with now feels like a factory. There is
no regard for me as an individual. I'm a uterus with so
many years behind it, that's all. It's an IVF clinic with a
good reputation and excellent statistics, but that's not
enough for me."

"If you talk to enough people you'll find a place that's
right for you. It's up to us to inform ourselves about the options," responds a soft-spoken woman in her forties. A wave
of agreement sweeps through the group. "Otherwise we're
just throwing our money away" comes a voice.

A petite brunette in a dark business suit takes charge of
the room: "I see so many people doing that. I guess infertility and weddings are two things people are willing to
throw tons of money at. Which is fine. Except that they are
willing to throw money at it and not learn about it. They
say, 'Oh, I'm gonna see this famous doctor. We're gonna

pay whatever it takes,' but that's not necessarily what gets you pregnant. Not that I know what gets you pregnant, but I do know I have to keep asking questions."

A man sitting two seats from me joins in: "And there are competent doctors out there who will listen. They won't be your therapists but they will do their job well. You can make an appointment just to talk to them." His wife, who is sitting next to him with one hand cupped over his, looks at him with such tenderness that for a moment I forget why I'm here and wish there was something I could do to help them. I also feel a pang of guilt, as if I were getting in line for seconds before everyone had been served.

After the support group, a presentation is scheduled in the room across the hall. Tonight's subject is the latest research on male infertility. I decide to stay just for a few minutes. A doctor from one of the leading medical centers in the tristate area is the key speaker. His introduction moves me: "There is a great deal in this field we still don't understand and are not sure about. At the same time, we are not comfortable with uncertainty, and so, we are constantly looking for reasons, for something to pick up." It's the first time since my diagnosis that I've heard a doctor say he is unsure about something.

The following day, I call his office. He is booked for the next few months, but one of his close associates, Dr. G, can see me in two weeks.

Sitting in Dr. G's waiting room, I wish I had brought her a small gift. Some symbol of goodwill. I think of my mother standing in the tiny garden in our backyard in

Kosice. She is cutting roses from her prized rosebush. She wraps the thorny stems in several layers of newspaper and carefully hands them to me. They are for my teacher, Mrs. Novak. My mother wants to connect with her. To thank Mrs. Novak for taking such good care of me.

I too want to connect with this woman doctor, thinking if she knew the person behind the chart it would deepen her desire to help me. It would inspire her to be more resourceful and to come up with the right combination of drugs.

The massive walnut desk covered with folders, the shelves packed with books, the framed diplomas hanging on the side wall; all the appropriate symbols of knowledge and authority add extra points to Dr. G's credibility. She's looking at my chart, nodding her head.

"You already have one child, that's good, but this is not so good," she says, pointing to the lab report with my latest FSH number. "I'm sorry, I wouldn't want to give you any false hope. This is not a good number. It means your ovaries are not working so well and unfortunately it gets worse with time. I'm afraid it's not something we could treat with medication or hormone drugs." She shrugs her shoulders and adds: "You're very lucky, there are lots of women out there who would love to be in your position."

After each of these appointments I hug Ellena a little tighter, I breathe her in more deeply. As we sit on our favorite stoop after morning errands, she with her bottle, I with my cup of coffee, I think I have the best life I could imagine. A minute later I get a hollow feeling in my belly,

as if I had committed some crime, but I can't quite remember what it is. I'm afraid that Ed and Ellena will have
to suffer the consequences. I'm afraid that what the experts
say is true, that there is nothing I can do. Seeking out more
specialists is for me the only way to fight back. If I see
enough of them, I'm bound to find one who will know
what to do.

My friend Lori shows up with the next instructions.
Lori and I worked in the same theater company for a couple of years, but we lost touch soon after I changed careers.
I vaguely remember a mutual friend mentioning that Lori
is having trouble getting pregnant. Now here she is, taking
over the sidewalk, in a sea of her favorite pastels, looking
like she is ready to walk onto the set of *The Umbrellas of
Cherbourg*. She is beaming.

First I get one of those long hard hugs one only gets
from actors. Then she spills the highlights of her infertility
in about twenty seconds. She had been trying to get pregnant for two years, she tells me. First they tried artificial
insemination for eight months. Her doctor was not very
optimistic, mainly because Lori had cervical cancer a few
years ago and had a lot of scar tissue. "Well, listen to this,"
she continues, trying to get the words out as fast as she can.
"After eight months with this quack, my aunt talked me
into flying out to Cleveland to see a specialist for a second
opinion. And you know what? He told me I was a perfect
candidate for pregnancy, my uterus was fine, and I would
have no problem carrying the baby. And you know what
else? He took one look at the lab reports from my old doc-

30   tor and in two seconds picked up the problem. He said that the sperm count of the sperm that came out of the lab was below the acceptable level. The lab was not processing the sperm well. As they were washing it, they were killing the sperm. He said, with these numbers, no wonder I'm not getting pregnant.

"I didn't know what those numbers meant. They sounded good enough to me. I vaguely remembered Andy's original sperm count being much higher than what was coming out of the lab. But it didn't really occur to me to question her competence. You expect them to be doing the right thing. I mean I didn't know she was a bad doctor. She went to good schools, she claimed she knew about infertility. I feel like marching around in circles in front of her office with a sign on my belly: 'If you want to look like me, stay away from this doctor.'

"By the way, if you know anybody who is looking for a specialist, the guy who helped me is great. Unfortunately, he's in Cleveland."

I am getting a little dizzy listening to Lori fast-forward through her story, but for the first time since my diagnosis, I am genuinely happy to hear about someone getting pregnant. Lori confirms my theory that the right doctor can make all the difference.

A few weeks later I call the doctor in Cleveland, and he spends twenty minutes on the phone with me, patiently answering all my questions. His colleague in New York can see me.

There are two empty seats in Dr. M's spacious Park Avenue waiting room. Sitting in a long line against the wall opposite the entrance are a young religious Jewish man in a gray-brimmed hat reading a prayer book, an Indian couple dozing on the sofa, and a young black woman holding an open textbook with a notepad. In the corner of the room, a young Muslim woman with traditional head covering lifts her enormous belly into a more comfortable position. Dr. M must have a contract with the United Nations. A sprinkling of other large bellies in the room tells me he is an obstetrician as well as a fertility expert, which is rare. As far as I know, the specialists usually take you through the first trimester and then send you off to an obstetrician.

Several sets of doors lead to examining rooms and what appears to be Dr. M's office. A nurse in scrubs smiles at one of the swollen bellies. "I'm ready for you, honey," she says. A few minutes later another blond nurse escorts a couple into Dr. M's office.

In one of the rooms off the narrow hallway, a saleswoman is selling pharmaceuticals. I pretend to examine the photographs of babies covering the wall and listen in. After all, she could have some relevant information. "This is the number-one safest allergy drug on the market," she says to a handful of nurses mulling around the room.

"Can pregnant women take it?" a nurse queries.

"Yes."

"Even in their first trimester?"

"Yes, absolutely. Only about four percent of the women may feel sedated and two percent may experience sleeplessness," assures the saleswoman.

A little while later I see her weaving through the rooms with a tray of small yellow boxes, like a hostess at a cocktail party. She offers a sample to the receptionist, then places a stack on the desk in Dr. M's office.

I have been here almost two hours, and the nurses are beginning to look familiar. A couple of them are chatting in Russian. Maybe I could put my thirteen years of compulsory Russian to good use, though I need to be careful. We foreigners don't always like it when strangers address us in our native language. I decide to play it safe and check on the state of affairs in English.

"Ms. Indichova?" she asks, expertly pronouncing my last name. "You're next."

"Something happened after your first child was born," says Dr. M, pacing the room as if trying to figure out what made my FSH surge so high. "I must say whatever it was, it happened awfully fast.

"I'm afraid I can't think of any current techniques that would reverse the damage. The only thing I can suggest is to take your levels every month and see if there's any significant change. You may also want to register with an IVF clinic, in case you decide to go that route." He hands me a sheet outlining a series of supplements that influence the reproductive system. B-complex, B, E, C, folic acid, calcium, zinc.

"Call me if your FSH comes down to at least the mid-twenties and we'll give Pergonal a try. I wish I could be more encouraging, but at this point I don't think anyone will be more optimistic," he adds, walking me to the door.

I do as the doctor says. For the next few months I take my supplements and monitor my FSH. The levels fluctuate between 35 and 40. I feel like I'm losing my footing. If only I could get my hand on a drug. So what if Dr. X, Y, or Z says it won't work? What if some unforeseeable set of circumstances will prove them wrong? A little Clomid, the aspirin of fertility drugs, couldn't do much harm. It would be something to do. I call Dr. C's nurse. "I'd like to try some Clomid this month," I say matter-of-factly, as if this were a choice outlined by the doctor.

Dr. C calls back. "Why don't we try a higher dosage this month?" he says.

"This is my first Clomid cycle," I answer. Clearly, he is not looking at my chart. Otherwise he would see that according to his diagnosis Clomid is not an option for me.

I get the stuff. I gulp it down as prescribed and wait. I keep touching my breasts. Are they getting sore, swelling up with life? Part of me feels like a kid who cheated on a test and made it to the elite group under false pretenses. I know sooner or later I'll be found out. I am. My period gives me away.

Up until now, whenever I needed help, my doctors told me what to do. But what do I do when they turn me loose?

Today, in the park I see a little girl on the bench next to ours. "Can I have some chewing gum?" she asks her mother.

34 "I'm sorry, I don't have any." The little girl turns toward Daddy. "Daddy, can I have some chewing gum?" she asks, holding on to his leg.

"I don't have any, Gillian."

That does not deter her from trying Grandma, who is out of chewing gum as well. I am a lot like that little girl. Bouncing off specialists, hoping the next one will give me what I want.

Dr. M is right. Whatever it is I'm after—a more hopeful prognosis, a pat on the shoulder, an earsplitting "Go, Julia!" it doesn't look like I'm going to get it. I'm a little worn out. My compulsion to search for the right answer is taking me away from Ellena and Ed. I keep telling myself how much I want this baby for them, but what they need right now is for me to stop drifting off into the infertility never-neverland.

We've been living in our three-room apartment since a month before Ellena's birth. Our original plan was to partition off part of the living room for her, but so far her crib is still in the corner of the living room, near our bedroom door. I jump up to check on her every time she stirs. Tonight, I hear her cough, and it sounds like a reproach. I want to do penance for my greediness and promise I'll stop wanting another baby as long as she is okay, as long as we're all healthy and safe.

In the morning I wake up with an image of the three of us sitting around the dining room table waiting for someone to show up. Loving each other deeply, but sad because someone is missing.

Aside from wanting to complete the family circle as I see it, other reasons might propel me to keep searching. I decided to give up acting a few years ago because at some point in my career each performance became a life and death situation. If I didn't live up to my high expectations, I felt my life was over. Between jobs all I did was obsess about whether or not I'd work again. Everything else was put on hold. Until one day I decided I could no longer live with that kind of pressure. I needed to get my life back and to know I was worthy without having to keep proving it onstage.

Now it looks like I'm back to proving I'm okay. And in order to do that I have to get pregnant again.

4

CHINESE
CHICKEN SOUP

When I grew up in Czechoslovakia in the 1950s, foreign countries looked like Hollywood movie sets where magic took place. Travel anywhere outside the Soviet satellite was restricted, and we had to curb our wanderlust in that political climate.

After twenty-four years of living in America, where I've been free to roam as far as my checkbook would take me, far-away places remain symbols of mystery and promise. After three months of Western medicine, I'm ready to leap all the way to China.

When I ask Dr. C what he thinks about using Chinese herbs to shake up my hormone levels, he replies without lifting his head from my chart: "There are certainly a lot of people in China. They must know something about making babies." Not quite the send-off into the world of Chinese medicine that I was hoping for, but my mind is made up.

I remember seeing a course on acupuncture in a New Age catalogue. The instructor's name is listed in the phone book. Mr. M, a practicing acupuncturist, can see me the next day.

His office is on the tenth floor of a commercial building. As I walk in, a slender man about my age, with dark brown hair and pale skin, speaks on the phone behind the reception desk. He nods in my direction, then continues to negotiate his dinner plans. "I just don't feel like anything elaborate. I think I'm coming down with something. Maybe we can just have a bowl of soup somewhere," he says, sounding like he should go straight to bed. Why can't he just put a few needles in his nose and drain the cold?

Without much preliminary dialogue he leads me toward the corner of the room, where a narrow massage table is separated by a white curtain. "I use disposable needles only," he says. I step on a small footstool and gingerly lower my body on the table. "Have you had acupuncture before?" he asks. I shake my head.

"There is nothing to be afraid of."

A moment later I feel a prick and a slight tingling sensation on the left side of my abdomen as he inserts the first needle.

Minutes later my entire body is decorated with needles, along the length of my legs, near my elbow and under my shoulder. One needle sticks out between my eyebrows, another from the crown of my head.

"Take nice long breaths and relax. We'll leave the needles in for about half an hour. I'll be back to check on you,"

38   he says, then pulls shut the curtain that separates me from the empty waiting room. The door to the hallway must be open as well; I hear footsteps going back and forth.

I can't say I'm entirely relaxed. My head has turned into a rare breed of porcupine and turning it to either side is unthinkable. I don't dare move my arms or legs. One of the points near my ankle feels very hot and tender. I have no idea where Mr. M is, or whether he would hear me if I called. Fortunately he does come back to check on me and adjusts a couple of the needles.

A little while later the needles are out, and we walk through a dark corridor into a small waiting room with four chairs lined up against the wall. A young Chinese couple and a woman with a teenage boy are waiting.

The acupuncturist leads the way to the alcove at the far end of the room. A smiling elderly Chinese woman in a white lab coat is filling Ziploc storage bags with little red berries, pieces of whitish tree bark shaped like tongue depressors, and what looks like debris that accumulates around dead tree trunks. She wraps each bag into a newspaper and hands over the packet to my acupuncturist.

"You are getting two sets of instructions. One is for making tea, the other one is for cooking the herbs with chicken. This will last you a couple of months," says Mr. M. He looks through his appointment book. "Should we make it the same time next week?" he asks, ready to write my name into the appropriate box.

"I'm not sure yet," I lie and flee for the nearest subway.

Maybe I was a little hasty about this appointment. The

next healer will be a referral by someone I trust. I ought to look for a doctor who has a deeper understanding of the medical system as well as the culture it grew out of. The next acupuncturist has to have a degree in Chinese medicine and—he has to be Chinese.

And Dr. R is. "How many days you have period? What is the color of blood? Pink?" she asks after I explain the purpose of my visit.

A small brown and gold velvet pillow serves as a resting place for my wrist while she takes my pulse, first on the right hand, then on the left. Her head drops forward, her short gray hair shading part of her cheeks.

"Kidney weak. Must make kidney strong. No needles for you, only build up the blood. In six months you pregnant. First make period more heavy, stronger body, warm up the blood, the blood must be warm to make baby." She walks to a large built-in closet: "Today in big city many people not healthy, many people eat in restaurant, in supermarket everything chemicals, if eat beef the farmers give it antibiotic and hormones to make it grow quicker. You eat hormones, no good, not natural." As she says this she opens the closet revealing hundreds of little plastic bags with tiny black and white balls. She selects four bags and hands them to me saying: "One day you take twelve white herbs, next day twelve black. You start first day after period."

She makes a note on a small index card and looks at me. "The red color is very strong color. You buy red sheets, bright red like this." She points to a silk shawl draped over the couch. "You only make love on red sheets."

40   Ellena would love to get her hands on the tiny black and white balls. She watches expectantly as I unwrap the newspaper and empty its mysterious contents into a large pot of water.

"I think the Jewish and the Chinese mothers made it up, they liked chicken, so they made it up, this thing about chicken soup being so good for you," says my Western husband as he sees me brewing a huge pot of twigs and barks floating around a feeble-looking chicken.

But we enjoy our new set of bright red flannel sheets, and I dutifully swallow my pellets. The sickly sweet smell of my tea and my new chicken soup doesn't much bother me. I like to suffer. It makes me feel like I'm paying my dues.

Yet something is missing. A part of me is sitting on the sidelines, saying: "Okay, sure, I'll do whatever you say. But you don't really expect me to believe in all this hocus-pocus."

The few books on Chinese medicine I leaf through at a local New Age bookstore might as well be written in Chinese. One of these days it might be time to grow up and do my own research, but right now I'm too anxious. I'm in a hurry.

I want someone who has already digested all the wisdom and will pass it on to me in a language I understand. Someone I can talk to. Someone with a family recipe, who could explain to me what my kidneys have to do with my high FSH. It seems the approach of each practitioner is unique.

Yet so far none of the healers has filled me with great confidence. I need to go further.

When my friend Lois mentions a Chinese doctor who has helped with afflictions Western doctors had given up on, I listen. "This woman I know," she says, when I share with her my ambivalence about Chinese medicine, "she had a sinus infection for twenty years, literally—the stuff coming out of her nose was black. She had a low-grade fever for a year, she went to Dr. B, and after five days the fever was gone. After two weeks the mucus was clear. Another woman was in her late thirties. She hasn't had her period in two years, and she went to Dr. B and in two months she started getting it again."

Testimonials like these are irresistible.

The doorman assumes an air of deference as he announces me through the intercom system. "Dr. B? Julia is on her way up."

As soon as I step out of the elevator, the scent of toasted tea leads me to the apartment at the end of the hall.

I'm greeted by an excited Pekingese and a young Chinese girl. She smiles, points to a chair in the hallway, and leaves. On the wall in front of me is a line of black and white photographs like the ones of Hollywood movie stars I collected as a child. One shows a young man in a white lab coat bending over a patient. Another is an autographed photo of Audrey Hepburn, which reads: "Thank you for being our fountain of youth."

I must have stumbled upon some well-kept secret that

only a privileged few have access to. The assistant escorts me to the living room. I am told to sit in an armchair facing the window.

"Where is your husband? He is not part of this?" says a voice behind me. Dr. B's face glides into my field of vision. He looks like someone who subsists solely on spring water, purified air, brown rice, and tofu. He could be forty, but he could also be sixty. His long bony body slowly unfolds into the armchair on the other side of the round coffee table.

"Is this your first experience with Chinese medicine?" he asks and something about his focused stare and the way he leans forward makes me lower my guard. I feel I can take all the time I need and tell him whatever I feel is important. When I give an account of my first acupuncture treatment, he responds with a story.

A peasant who had worked as a laborer in a Western missionary hospital decided, after his retirement, to take some hypodermic needles back to his village. He also packed a large supply of antibiotics. When he got home he put up a shingle, and pretty soon the word about his wonder drugs spread throughout the region. He cured many of his patients in spite of the fact that he knew nothing about Western medicine.

"Maybe your acupuncturist has something in common with this peasant. Acupuncture can be strong medicine, even if you don't understand why," he says.

He asks me a few basic questions about my medical history, my first pregnancy and delivery. All of this reinforces my confidence in him.

In the middle of the room is a long table. I lie down on it fully clothed, and Dr. B starts bending, then straightening, first my arms and then my legs, as if he were checking for broken limbs. Then he asks me to pull up my legs into a cross-legged position and swing my body to the right, so that now I am sitting sideways in the middle of the narrow part of the table. He stands behind me and asks me to lower my body backward. "Just relax and let your body hang," he says, holding my back to support me.

Next he presses down on my abdomen, then helps me sit back up and palpitates all along my spine. "I'm probing your back for energy blockage," he says. Sensing my need to know more, he explains how the Chinese medical system is based on a belief that an energy, called Qi (pronounced *chee),* permeates the entire universe. It flows through our bodies along pathways called meridians.

"If this energy becomes blocked we get sick. When we get sick, our balance of yin and yang is affected. You must know about yin and yang?" Without waiting for a response he continues. "Yang is fire. Yin is water. Yang is masculine, yin is feminine. Yang is light, yin is dark. Our job is to bring yin and yang into balance."

A consultation and a crash course in Chinese medicine, I think, feeling encouraged. "Why are you looking at my ears?" I ask when he starts bending and scrutinizing the cartilage. "The veins on your ears tell me a great deal about your hormone levels. The kidneys are the *root of life.* They rule birth, development, and reproduction. There is a close relationship between the kidneys and the ears."

44   He is pressing down on several points on my back, commenting as he goes along. "Your muscles are very tight. They block the flow of energy. I'm doing acupressure on your back to help open up the muscles and the flow of blood.

"I can't find any reason why you would not be able to have a baby. There is nothing wrong with you," he says finally.

Isn't this what I came for? A clean bill of health? Why don't I feel relieved?

Dr. B tells me to take notes.

"The pulse that relates to your digestive system is a little weak. When your digestive system is weakened, you don't process things well and the whole movement of energy from the top to the bottom can be disturbed. I will give you some herbal formulas to help with that kind of stagnation."

He brings out a rectangular cardboard box with Chinese writing and a red and black drawing of a chicken. He opens the box and takes out a wax ball. Inside the ball are lots of tiny black pellets similar to the ones I'm already taking. "This is a gentle but nourishing formula that will build up your blood and your energy. One of the few herbal formulas made from chicken. You can get a refill in a Chinese pharmacy.

"Next thing, foods. Eat a lot of soups. They are easier to digest. Also, I want you to go to Chinatown and look for *dhuri* fruit. It's very high in protein. You would be surprised how many *dhuri* babies are running around in this city. You should eat only warm foods, nothing cold, no cold drinks, no ice cream. You have too much cold in you. Apple cinnamon tea is a nice warming tea."

He continues, "Vitamin E is the magic vitamin. Take 400 milligrams twice a day. To improve your circulation, take hot and cold showers every morning and every evening. You'll turn on the cold water, count to five then make the water as hot as you can stand and count to five again. You do this six times. Jumping rope will also help with your circulation. It makes your organs shake. If your organs shake, they get stronger. Without exercise your muscles weaken, not just your muscles but your organs as well. You should do three hundred jumps a day.

"Most importantly, you need to keep asking yourself why you want this baby so much. Do you want it for yourself, to own it, so you can say you have two children? Or is it to be a channel of your love to send out into the universe?"

"Oh, yes," I say quickly. "A channel of my love for Ed and Ellena."

My time is up. As I reach for my purse he discreetly motions toward a small ceramic bowl where I am to leave my hundred and fifty dollars in cash.

"If you are not pregnant in six months, call me." He walks out the door.

Two days later, Ed looks around the kitchen. "What's that smell?" he asks.

"Don't touch it, it's very sharp," I call out in warning as he examines the large thick brown ball covered with needles in the middle of the counter.

46 As a fruit, *dhuri* leaves something to be desired. As a medieval weapon, however, it could be quite effective. The smell is a cross between the aged cheese my father used to bring out when he wanted to hasten the departure of our guests and a refrigerator that needs cleaning. If one can somehow ignore the smell, the taste is actually not bad at all. The soft fleshy insides could pass for a cantaloupe.

It took a great deal of investigation to find one of the few stores in Chinatown that carries it. I paid twelve dollars for the smallest specimen on display. That included getting it cut open, which could have been life-threatening. The first *dhuri* lasted a few days, and I could only bring myself to repeat the experience one more time.

Next, hot and cold showers are the toughest part of Dr. B's regime. But I take them twice a day.

I do a pretty good impersonation of an exemplary patient. I even decide to get a refill on the herbs from Dr. B for my third month. I brew tea and cook chicken. The sweet smoky mist that hovers over the apartment and seeps through my clothes is almost pleasant. But my mind is tightly clenched. I can't quite make the connection between the herbs, my kidneys, and my FSH.

Maybe it's cultural. If my mother had depended on twigs and barks to cure my colds, I might be more open to using them now.

The truth is, I expected an instant cure. An herb, an acupuncture point that would bring on an instant change. Turn my menstrual blood into a healthy piercing pink and make it flow freely for five long days. Sadly, my body is not cooperating.

I understand that the imbalances in my body, which have taken forty-two years to accumulate, will not disappear overnight. I understand that Chinese medicine is not about immediate results and powerful drugs. I deeply respect the holistic approach to illness that informs the Chinese medical system. But after three months, I can't bring myself to swallow any more herbs, and I need a break from the cold showers.

Who knows? Maybe the little white balls and the funky chicken soup have already made their mark, even if I don't feel or see any change.

5

GETTING IN LINE

A beloved acting teacher used to tell us to always schedule something fun to do after an important audition. He said it would save us the agony of waiting for a callback and help us get on with our lives.

I follow his advice when it comes to important doctors' appointments, which means I have a busy week planned. We're in the waiting room of one of the highest-rated IVF clinics in the world.

For most couples who have trouble conceiving, the descent into the infertility underworld is gradual. It starts out with a few cycles of Clomid, through artificial insemination, cycles of Pergonal, and finally, at the bottom, is the entrance to the IVF clinic. Sometimes it takes years to hit all the sights. But my FSH pushed me right to the front of the line in less than six months.

It seems odd that less than six months ago words such as

adoption, surrogacy, and *infertility* were headlines on the covers of women's magazines that briefly crossed my field of vision at the supermarket checkout counter. They had nothing to do with me.

When the Russians invaded Czechoslovakia in 1968 and women from the nearby village hurried through the streets with arms full of candles, bread, and canned food, I suddenly found myself in the middle of a World War II movie. The tanks rolled in firing shells in the air, and my father, terrified by the sound, pulled me to the ground. I couldn't just close my eyes and wait for the scary part to be over. It was real.

This, too, is real. This is Ed and I sitting in a waiting room of a hospital because we can't get pregnant on our own. Yet we can't afford to stand still.

We give our name to the receptionist and wait. After about twenty minutes I get a little restless. I'm aware that one ought to be prepared to wait in a doctor's office well beyond one's scheduled appointment. But the clinic called me only yesterday to fill in for a last-minute cancellation, and I was assured that the doctor would be on time. I need to get to my class at Hunter College in a couple of hours.

The receptionist ignores us. We are the only couple here, but she is on the phone, negotiating the repair of her Volvo.

Ordinarily, this would be a perfect opportunity to practice a well-controlled, articulate expression of anger. But I'm too anxious. I timidly walk up to the desk and apologize for interrupting her. (She is now talking to her sister about a possible weekend lunch date with Mom.) I politely ask how much longer she thinks we have to wait.

She puts her hand over the receiver and shrugs. "It shouldn't be much longer." Then she quickly returns to the phone, not wanting to lose her train of thought.

After an hour's wait, we decide that waiting any longer will cut our appointment to a less-than-useful time. We gather our belongings and tell the receptionist we're leaving. As we walk toward the exit the doctor appears, her arm extended for a handshake.

I explain my time consideration, and she assures me I'll be done in forty-five minutes. But she seems irritated that we dared to challenge the order of things by announcing our departure. "If you can't trust us enough to know that we do our best, maybe this is not the right place for you."

This makes me totally lose my cool, and I start crying. "I know, usually I'm prepared to wait, but . . ."

Her tone changes. "Sorry, I'll have to have a word with the staff. They should never promise something like that. Why don't we just go over your records and sort through some of your options. If need be, we will do the physical exam at another time," she says slowly, as if to let us know there's plenty of time. She is about my age. Her white coat is open, making her appear less formal. Underneath it she is wearing a brick-colored cotton sweater and a pair of comfortable slacks. I wonder if she has children, and if she gets to be with them as much as she would like to.

I hand over copies of my lab reports and tell her my story. She agrees with the recommendations of the referring specialist. Monitoring my FSH may be a good idea, but she also thinks that this high a number indicates a radical decline in my ovarian function. Sadly, there are no pleasant surprises in her doctor's kit, no fresh-off-the-slide breakthroughs. "We can only work with you in our egg donor program," she says. "Doing anything else would simply not be in your best interest. We want to do all we can to maximize your chances of success."

This is pretty much what we expected, but I was secretly hoping to use my own eggs if the FSH dropped.

Ed is ready with questions. "How do you find your donors?"

She answers, as she must have many times before: "Mostly we advertise, and some of our donors hear about us through word of mouth. There are two basic types of donors. Students in their early to mid-twenties who need the money, and also they feel it's a neat thing to do. Or they are mothers in their early thirties who had a relative or a friend with fertility problems, and they want to help."

I want to know how long it usually takes to find a suitable donor. Dr. S shows us the application form, several pages long. "It depends on what is important to you and how flexible you are about your requirements. Some couples come in wanting a Harvard graduate, preferably in a doctoral program, who is a virtuoso flute player," she says, laughing a little to show she is only half serious. "But mostly we would look for someone to match Julia's coloring, then have the person go through a series of interviews with one of our doctors, as well as a psychologist. If all goes well, the next step is taking a thorough medical history."

Ed wants to know if we could find someone ourselves. "Oh, sure, many people do," she says. "We would still screen them. And we do have a cap on age. We don't accept any donors over thirty-five."

I try to imagine a hospital room with two stretchers lined up side by side. I'm lying on one of them. A carefree, sophomoric face smiles at me from the other. A syringe filled with a quivering row of freshly retrieved eggs is being passed down from one gloved hand to the next. "Can you tell us how the actual procedure works?" I ask, thinking this may be a slightly distorted picture.

"We start by turning off the cycles of both women with Lupron. Then we synchronize them. The donor is given hormones to boost her egg production, and Julia would take some simple medication to duplicate the course of her menstrual cycle. The eggs are retrieved from the donor and fertilized the same day. Three or four embryos are then transferred into Julia's uterus. It takes two weeks to see if the procedure has worked."

She hands us a folder with lots of reading material and adds, "This is a step-by-step outline of everything you need to know. You can always call me if you have further questions. But I would like you to stop in to see our psychologist before you go."

The long, flowing skirt of the staff psychologist makes her look out of place among all the white lab coats with little picture IDs pinned to breast pockets. She is one of us, a civilian.

"My part in all this is to help you decide whether or not

this is right for you. There are a lot of things to work through," she says. She has been alerted about our time constraint and is prepared with a few take-home assignments: "You have to come to terms with Julia's losing a biological link to the baby. And that's something for both of you to work on."

She turns to Ed. "When you got married, you thought you were going to have children with Julia, but this baby will not have her genes."

I wonder if Ed is thinking, as I am, how much more devastating this would be if we didn't have Ellena. "You need to think about whether or not you tell the child how he or she came to you, or whether you keep it closed." She runs her fingers through her shortly cropped hair, and leans against the back of her chair.

There is a great deal more for us to talk about, but my students are waiting. "Call if you have questions. You can even come by and see me again if you need to. I'm sorry this appointment was more stressful than it should have been," she says sympathetically.

Ed speed-walks me to the subway. "We will have another baby," he says. "We'll fight our way to her or him, no matter what it takes." He hugs me and hails a cab. Watching the taxi swerve into traffic, knowing what the three hours away from his desk will do to his day, I feel a familiar pang of guilt. There is never a trace of blame in his behavior toward me. But he is hurting, because I let him down.

On the subway ride to work I think about the first time the two of us talked about getting married. "The only thing

54   is," said Ed, "we'd have to have children right away. You are older."

I am. Exactly six and a half years older than Ed. I was thirty-eight when we met, thirty-nine when we got married. He wanted children, his own family. He took a chance on me. Now he is paying for it.

After the years of roommates, blind dates, relationships that were supposed to be "good for me," he came into my life just in the nick of time. Just when everyone was ready to give up on me.

"You know, you don't really have to get married," said my cousin, the mother of two gorgeous boys. "Why put yourself under that kind of pressure? Not everybody has to have children." But I wanted them. I wanted to have children. What a fool I was, pretending even to myself that it would be okay not to, because I wasn't sure I'd ever meet someone to have them with.

"This is Ed, Eddie? I met you at Fire Island last weekend," he said the first time he called me.

I met him at the sunset party in Fair Harbor, a vacation spot for singles. I was standing with a cup of hot tea in my hand, setting myself apart from all those calculating single women with real drinks. Oh, no, not me, I'm just hanging out. I'm back in graduate school working on getting a teaching license. I don't need a man to pump meaning into my life.

Strategically dressed in white to offset my tan, no bra. Noticing from the corner of my eye all the flirting around me. Then a face. A light, gentle face. Is he talking to me? "Excuse me, I saw you dancing at the Dock a couple of weeks ago. You're a great dancer," he says in an even-tempered voice. He looks much too handsome. Light brown hair, high cheekbones, blue-green eyes. He's obviously not Jewish, though I don't think anyone in my family would really care at this point. Five years ago they might have groaned. But this is the eleventh hour. Now my family sees me as a *bovlie,* a Yiddish word for merchandise that sits on the shelf.

Still, he looks too young. I better clear this up right away. "How old are you?" I ask provocatively.

"Thirty-two. How old are you?"

"Thirty-eight." That should be enough to have him make a graceful exit. But he's not moving.

"Do you speak another language?" he asks, hearing my accent.

"I speak a few other languages," I reply, not wanting to make this too easy for either one of us.

A few more chess moves, then: "Would you like to go dancing sometime?"

We walk back to the weekend house I share with five other women to get a paper and pen. He has a sweet, open face. I'm a little nervous. I want him to like me. It seems he already does.

All of my roommates happen to be home. His exit is a cue for a curious chorus: "How did you meet him? He said that? Oh, how sweet. What does he do? Very cute, very, very cute."

"You're crazy, he's too young for me," I say, thinking he may never call.

"You know, you both have great cheekbones. You could have gorgeous kids, you two," says Patricia, hugging her fifteen-year-old daughter.

And, in just a skip of time, we do. Our angel of angels, Ellena. If I can't rally into action on my own behalf, I must get moving for her and for Ed. But it is going to take work.

The stream of play dates we scheduled for this week helps. Ellena has a new pal in the building. She and Eric became fast friends the moment we met him and his father, Ted, in our lobby. Eric and Ellena took one look at each other, burst out laughing, and ran to a cozy corner under the stairwell, where they continued to chuckle and play for another five minutes.

Eric's parents, Ted and Merrill, have been enormously helpful in the last couple of months. They've offered to share their baby-sitter, which means if I need to, I can leave for work before Ed gets home. Merrill often takes care of Ellena during my early morning doctors' appointments.

Holding on to my daughter's small hand, I commute from the city of playgrounds and baby bottles to the underground city of IVF clinics and hysterosalpingograms that shoot a dye into your fallopian tubes. You shut your eyes tight, squeeze your husband's hand, and wait for the dye to rise—slowly—then strike the deepest, most tender place inside you.

A Slovak idiom comes to mind when I reflect on my emotional state of the last few months. *Uzko mi je* literally translates as *It's narrow in me.* During my adolescence it meant a kind of quiet dread of an upcoming event, a feeling of deep uncertainty. When I think of it now, I feel a narrowness in my chest, a constriction that keeps me from taking a deep breath. I think of impersonal narrow corridors, leading to examining rooms. I think of narrow lovemaking zeroed in on the one thing that's unattainable.

I realize how afraid I am to open up to the sadness, afraid to let Ed see. It seems like such an ungrateful, foolish thing to feel in the midst of all the astounding good luck I have already been showered with.

I must keep moving. I can't just sit around agonizing over my options while my childbearing days gallop away from me. I must fight against all the grave faces that say it's useless—all these appointments, all this flapping of my wings.

Though we are not sure about going the egg-donor route, in the weeks following the consultation with Dr. S, Ed and I go over our Rolodex of fertile, generous, brilliant, and beautiful friends under thirty-five.

Most of our friends fit all but one of the requirements. Even if they're under thirty-five today, in a week or two we would have to scratch them off the list. We could lie. They all look under thirty-five. But no, that's bad karma.

It's definitely slim pickings in the egg department, but we do have some choices.

"My friend George, he has great kids and his wife, Jane, is very sweet. I bet she'd do it for us," says my resourceful husband. "And you know who else? Beth. She would be totally into it. She felt bad when I told her we were having trouble."

"Bad enough to get injected with Pergonal twice a day for two weeks and then lose a handful of eggs?" I ask, feeling less than optimistic.

"Maybe," he says.

Even if we found a donor, I'm not ready to do IVF anytime soon. But I don't know how I will feel six months or a year from now. So I might as well go through all the requisite tests and get in line. It's like taking a number at the crowded deli counter at Zabar's, even though you're not sure you will use it.

I also decide to follow Dr. G's recommendation to keep monitoring my FSH. The clinic does blood tests every morning, including weekends. That means that two days after I get my period, I head to the East Side for my day-three FSH test. After each of these early morning excursions, my head is alight with fragments of conversations particular to IVF clinic waiting rooms: "We are stopping Pergonal. I have a cyst on my ovaries, we have to wait until it comes down." Or: "My doctor doesn't recommend doing it more than three times. But I met a woman at a Resolve meeting who did it twelve times, and finally, she got pregnant."

Everyone in the room has either heard of someone to whom IVF has given one, or two, maybe even three babies; or of someone else who had gone through every high-tech procedure and didn't get pregnant.

One morning I walk into the clinic's bathroom and hear what sounds like an impromptu consciousness-raising group. A young woman with curly red hair is wiping her eyes: ". . . and when I started crying, the nurse said I shouldn't give up, that the doctor would let us know when it was time to give up hope. I was reeling. Who the hell made him the Lord High Keeper of Hope?"

A woman standing at the sink next to her shakes her head and sighs. "They are very encouraging with us. In a way I wish they would find something wrong. But everything checks out. That's why I can't give up. If there is nothing wrong, then one day it's got to work."

Most of the time I'm afraid to join in the conversation, thinking my motherhood disqualifies me from being a true member. But one morning at the clinic I find myself sitting next to Nancy, a woman about my age, who after a few exchanges turns to me and says, "I have a five-year-old at home who keeps asking me why he can't have a brother or a sister." Nancy tells me secondary infertility is quite common.

"We go to a Resolve support group once a week," she says. "It's very helpful. Let me give you my number, in case you'd like to check it out." I take the number and thank her, moved by her openness. But I'm still not ready for a support group. That would make everything even more real.

I look at the faces of the women and men around me and I see all the grown-up social masks washed away by fear. Instead of a roomful of adults, we are children. We've been called on the carpet, and we don't know why. Nor do we know what our punishment will be.

On a small table next to the receptionist's desk lies a sign-up sheet filled with names. Next to the name is the first day of each woman's menstrual cycle and the test she needs to have done. The cumulative anxiety, pain, hope, and expectation of all those names fills the room. If only we could transform all that feeling into a giant force, the strength of our joint intention could surely bring forth a baby a day. We would meet here every morning, the woman whose turn it was would sit in the center of the circle, surrounded by a chain of our hands, a wall of giving, until we each got our turn. "And don't forget you're here for seconds," whispers a voice in my head.

To think there was a time when all we had to do was make love. Seven months after we got married (how foolish of us to waste those precious seven months!), it was time to pack away my diaphragm and go into production. Ed was taking classes for his certificate in computer programming in the evening, and during the day he worked on his computer at home. On crucial days I whisked into a cab on my lunch hour and rushed home for one more round of production, to make sure that little egg got plenty of prospective sperms to choose from.

There were no third parties, no post-coital tests, no hormone levels, no biopsies of my uterus. Just a little extra lovemaking, followed by the voice of a lab technician I briefly chatted with when I went for my pregnancy test: "You know, I'm not supposed to be the one to tell you this, you'll officially hear it from your doctor, but I couldn't wait. It looks like you're pregnant."

Now there is a squadron of assistants. Doctors, psychologists, advisers. Endless procedures. Shiny metal instruments prodding inside me, looking to see if anything else is wrong.

Lying in bed at night I strain to screen out the multitude of voices, but in spite of all my resolve to move forward, I'm losing touch with my body and slipping back into despair.

Perhaps I need to remind myself how far I have come

from the bad old days. The eight years of coming home to my empty one-room studio apartment, with the fluctuation of my self-esteem directly proportionate to the number of male messages on my answering machine. The days of my various temp jobs that were meant to keep me afloat financially until my big break in the theater. The frustrating tango of my acting career. Of coming inches away from success, then quickly drawing back from it.

To have put all the fear and self-torture of those days behind me is a miracle.

What about the incredible luck of marrying Ed, instead of one of the hot prospects that wanted to remake me in his own Ivy League image? What about the astounding good fortune of being Ellena's mom?

I should make a list of all my blessings and carry it in my pocket to ward off sadness.

In spite of all my doubts, it seems I have completed the prerequisite round of testing. My hysterogram confirms that my tubes are open and willing. Several other tests show I am a perfect candidate for an egg-donor IVF.

Today a small packet arrives in the morning mail to commemorate my full membership in the world of technologically assisted conception. It contains a series of prescriptions for hormonal medications, two syringes, and a diagram of instructions on how to administer the twice daily injections of Pergonal. I can barely look at any of it. How will I ever be brave enough to use it?

6

CLEANING THE REFRIGERATOR

One's destination is never a place but rather
a new way of looking at things.

—HENRY MILLER

It has been almost nine months since the alarming news of my high FSH. The medical community tells me there is nothing I can do, other than shop around for some fertilizable eggs. Alternative healers are optimistic, but, as far as I can tell, none of their suggestions have brought me any closer to my goal. So far we've been lucky to afford our quest for the miracle treatment. Though lately, we've been dipping into our savings and the pile of unpaid bills on my desk warns me to withdraw temporarily from any more consultations.

Something else has happened. With Ellena eating more solid foods, I've been reading more closely the nutritional content and ingredients on boxes of cereals, crackers, cookies, pasta, jars of tomato sauce, and other staples. My loyalty has gradually shifted from the supermarket to the health food store, and since most days I don't leave for work until the late afternoon, Ellena and I often browse around at Health Nuts.

Her blue eyes and her babyhood attract a great deal of attention from the staff. Dorgyi, a sweet-mannered man from Tibet, laughs warmly as soon as he sees us come in. If he has the time, he comes over, lifts her out of the stroller, and takes her on a tour of the produce section, or walks over to the frozen-yogurt machine behind the deli counter and gives her a taste of "ice" in a tiny paper cup.

Theresa, who has the bearing and looks of a European movie star, glides through the aisles in her long flowery skirt. *"Czesc,* Ellenka," she says in Polish, using the Slavic diminutive of her name.

Today, as any other day, Ellena clamors for every package of chips and cookies within reach. Luckily, Jay, the manager, walks by with a cracker and a high five.

While Ellena holds court at the deli counter, I have a few minutes to browse through the variety of titles at the book section. Many of the authors suggest that diet can profoundly affect the body's ability to heal itself and change its overall energy. What I read seems to relate directly to my tired body, and to my ovaries, which allegedly can no longer produce fertilizable eggs. As I stand in the narrow aisle between the brown rice crackers and the books, I begin to think, Can *I* do anything to help myself? Can *I* possibly be capable enough to launch a research project of my own? Look for answers within these books? What I eat must affect the way my body functions. How could it not?

64   Ever since I can remember, the taste and smell of my favorite foods have been my loyal companions. One mouthful of poppy-seed noodles, cheese dumplings, sausage and onions, and I'm home again, listening to my mother shuffle around in the kitchen on a Sunday morning.

The events of the past year have only cemented my emotional reliance on food. To paraphrase one of my favorite Shakespeare sonnets: "and each of my moods hath its adjunct morsel/wherein it finds comfort above the rest."

My best strategy for dealing with another disappointing consultation is to wolf down the largest piece of chocolate cake money can buy. Waiting for results of another FSH test is more manageable over a plate of chicken (ideally, my mother's chicken paprikash recipe). The sound of a friend's less than sympathetic remark, when you tell her you may not be able to have another child, fades in the steam of a cappuccino. A range of unpleasant incidents is erased by a large quantity of food consumed at great speed.

I remember a colleague of mine, years ago, frustrated with his young son's eating. "I tell him the body is like an intricate, finely tuned machine. If you don't take care of it, if you stuff it with junk—it breaks."

Most of the books at the health food store talk about the importance of proper digestion and elimination. Many recommend less meat, eating whole grains, raw and cooked vegetables, a variety of beans, and foods that contain omega-3 fatty acids. They also agree it's better to substitute desserts made from sweet vegetables, like squash or sweet potatoes, for desserts made with refined sugar.

It sounds too virtuous, not to mention restrictive. Yet, didn't the last Chinese doctor I saw tell me my digestive system was weakened? I stopped taking the little black pellets he gave me, but maybe working on my diet can be as effective. After three weeks of reading, it becomes clear that I need to simplify my diet, use some self-discipline and eat foods that will supply me with nutrients, not empty calories. If I lighten the work of the digestive system, there will be more energy left for rejuvenation.

I become intensely aware of my usually unconscious eating. It's amazing how indiscriminately my hand travels toward my mouth with just about anything it can find. If it's within reach and even remotely edible, in it goes. A bite of banana left on the high chair, trails of Cheerios, a piece of chicken that happens to cross my field of vision as I open the refrigerator, little surprises left under the couch pillows. You'd think my jaws would be sore from all that chewing. I'm certainly not hungry. But am I giving all those billions of hungry little cells what they need? Are my wilting ovaries energized by stale Cheerios?

Maybe I haven't been treating my body as well as I can. Maybe it's asking me to strike up a bargain. You want something from me? Well, it will cost you. Do you realize I hardly ever get a fair share of greens? Or fruit? That often days go by without any grains? You're gonna have to do a little better.

The first thing I adapt is what several of the diet plans refer to as the principles of natural hygiene. Nothing but fruit and juices till noon, to give the body a chance to cleanse itself.

66   My initial fears of caffeine and buttered croissant withdrawal are unfounded. This is not that difficult. Adah, my
Israeli friend, is unimpressed. "That's how I've always been
eating." Radiant, energetic Adah, the mother of two gorgeous boys.

The transition is eased, fueled by my desire. I'm on a
mission. I find myself leaning toward several other ideas.

Although a vegetarian diet has made sense to me for
years, I didn't see myself as disciplined enough to follow
one. Chicken, turkey, and eggs were good, wholesome
home cooking to me. I viewed vegetarians as belonging to
one of two groups: either a radical, fundamentalist sect,
whose members police local restaurants armed with leaflets
full of bean sprout propaganda, or a less intrusive subgroup,
spiritual, transcendent, globally informed, well read and
written. My friend Allen is a member of the second, subsisting in his East Village apartment on millet and adzuki
beans, typing away at his manuscript, refusing to become a
cog in the capitalist machine.

But since my consciousness with regard to meat has not
been concerned with the ethical and moral implications of
diet, there seemed no need to follow a meatless path. Now
I want my body to give me something, and I am willing to
do just about anything in return. If it's a choice between a
hamburger and a baby, I'll take the baby.

Ed is game to try anything. He is a graduate of the CIA
(Culinary Institute of America), and before switching to
computer programming, he worked as a professional chef at

several of the finest French restaurants in New York. Under his guidance, I expand my repertoire of dishes. Sunday afternoon, we're at the two cutting boards, while Ellena plays with the Legos on the kitchen floor. We're prepping for tonight's cauliflower and carrot casserole. Ed is once again showing me how to cut vegetables without sprinkling them with freshly drawn blood.

"When you're holding the carrots, curve your fingers so the knife rests against the knuckles," he says. "Let the knife do the work, back and forth. Slice, don't chop."

My husband is a calming influence in my life, and his presence in the kitchen is no exception. For the first time, I am happy to be learning how to cook. No more temperamental chefs like my ex-roommates, barking orders and shrieking over burnt rice.

"If you cut the cauliflower through, it crumbles. But if you just cut the stem and pull it apart, it breaks along the natural lines." He holds out a perfect floret to Ellena, who is tiring of Legos and clamoring for a bottle.

"Nyam, I want nyam," she screams until Ed picks her up and hands her a butter knife. Cutting up tofu is her job, since it doesn't require a sharp knife or force. But she isn't in the mood today.

Ed makes a bottle with a couple of ounces of juice, trying to stall her till dinner. She's not happy. "Big nyam! I want big nyam!" she shouts as Ed carries her out of the kitchen.

The menu for the rest of the week features tempeh with

soy sauce, honey, and a touch of sesame oil; broccoli sautéed with olive oil and minced garlic; chickpeas and rice; lentil soup; and salads. For desserts, we titillate the palate with a well-loved banana pudding, adzuki-almond mousse, or cookies from Health Nuts.

The next step is the weaning of my dairy dependence. It's not easy, but the rewards are quick.

I have become so accustomed to the discomfort of my sinus headaches that they seem a part of me. I spend many an evening with my thumb and index finger pressing down on the bridge of my nose to relieve the pressure. The notion that dairy products might be to blame is quite alien, un-American.

Yet several publications claim that some people develop allergies to milk and milk products. I recall one of the Chinese doctors warning me against the residues of hormones and drugs used on some modern farms.

I experiment with a variety of rice- and almond-based drinks.

Three weeks later, I develop what appears to be a bad cold. I can't stop blowing my nose. Where is all this thick white mucus coming from? And why don't I feel sick? I have no other cold symptoms. I must be just getting unclogged. My sinuses are a lot clearer and—I can hardly believe it—my headaches are gone.

In moments of weakness, my legs carry me into Vinnie's Pizzeria. Like a junkie looking for a fix, I reach for what I know to be the best slice on this side of the Atlantic. That generous triangle of "extra cheese and pepperoni" can be as satisfying as curling up under Grandma's blanket on a rainy Sunday. But these days, it feels too much like I'm doing myself in. So I do what my friend Leila learned in her eating-disorder support group: I take a bite and get rid of the rest.

A month later, I'm rewarded when the first vegetarian pizzeria in New York opens a few blocks from my house. They offer everything from spelt, corn, and whole-wheat crust to tofu toppings with organic vegetables. They even make a rice pudding with brown rice and almond milk. It's a sign: Somebody up there is cheering me on!

Although we've made major changes in our diet, I can't say we're following a particular regimen. For example, Ellena now drinks rice milk, organic goat and cow's milk, and she loves yogurt. We no longer eat meat, but we still eat fish, and we use organic eggs for baking. For the time being I've stopped all dairy products.

By the third month, the diet adjustments become easier, as if my body is saying, "Hey, what took you so long?" Not only do I not feel that I am giving something up, I realize I am finally taking care of myself. Maybe that is what this baby wants, a mother who knows how to be her own mother first.

Aside from the one cycle of Clomid, I haven't taken any fertility drugs. The IVF clinic prescriptions lie untouched in the back of my file cabinet. Yet, once in a while, I'm tempted to try just one more specialist. Part of me is still hoping to come upon someone with the right credentials to tell me FSH levels don't mean much.

Dr. K's name is connected with many success stories, and my insurance covers the cost of the visit. As soon as I cite my particular numbers, his eyebrows go up, his face grows solemn, a sigh, a handshake, and I'm on my own. Nothing has changed.

My friend Allen tries cheering me up: "What's the difference between a doctor and God?" he asks. After a slight pause: "God doesn't think he is a doctor." I'm usually so anxious about rewarding Allen's jokes with a sufficiently buoyant response that I rarely get their meaning, but this one hits the spot.

As time goes by, my faith in the godliness of doctors fades. I struggle to replace it with the confidence that my body knows what's best for it. It's telling me that if I keep listening, keep working, I can strengthen it enough to bring forth life again.

This is the most difficult part, this pivotal leap of faith. After all, I have never questioned medical authorities, never interfered with their ministrations, doubted their omniscience. Shaking myself free of their certainty takes will. Close my eyes. Grit my teeth. Do more research.

The slightest movement on the horizon brings hope. A food, an herb, a healer. A snippet of conversation overheard in a restaurant gets me out of my chair: "Excuse me, what was the book you mentioned?" I ask.

My class at Hunter College ends at nine-thirty, and most nights, I don't get home until ten-thirty. Ed leaves for work at six in the morning, which means he is often asleep by the time I get back.

The night silence is irresistible. I splash cold water on my face and make a cup of tea. The two books I picked up at Health Nuts this morning are sitting next to the toaster. A chance to settle in for an hour or two of uninterrupted work is too precious to squander on sleep.

The bathroom happens to be the only place in the apartment where the reading light won't disturb the rest of the household. There I sit on our lovely black and white tiles, stocking up on words that will lower my FSH.

Louise Tenney's *Health Handbook* lists beans, peas, raw nuts, and seeds under fertility boosters. Someone mentions the importance of diuretic foods, such as cucumber and watermelon, in renewing hormonal balance. The iodine in seaweed is said to have the same balancing effect. Mana, my favorite macrobiotic restaurant, serves burdock—revered as an excellent source of vitamins and minerals—in a delicious ginger sauce. It's a beginning. I start eating these foods.

Friends and relatives offer home remedies and family anecdotes. My aunt Lilli in Florida says, "You must gain weight, you're too thin," or "A glass of red wine at night will help build up your blood." A coworker who follows a macrobiotic diet has heard that a carrot-daikon drink with seaweed and umeboshi will help with female hormonal problems. Ed's cousin Annie tells me of a study in Boston in which women who added a certain number of bagels to their diet increased their ability to conceive. I love bagels, but I find it a little hard to see them as pulsating with life-giving nutrients. I hold off on any radical shift in my bagel consumption.

My friend Karen, an herbologist and tree lover, sends me a nurturing package of herbs and tinctures: nettles to build up my iron, oatstraw for calcium, licorice to stimulate estrogen production, milk thistle seed extract to support better liver function.

Slowly yet steadily, over a period of three months, my entire relationship to food is changing. All I want from it is to make me stronger, cleaner, more energetic. I had been perfectly content to have some "bad" stuff, as long as I balanced it with enough "good" food. Gradually, I've come to eliminate anything that might be even remotely harmful. If it's not going to be useful, I don't want it.

In addition to clearer sinuses, my stomach has never felt better. Ed, the ultimate encourager, has also changed his eating habits, and is now trumpeting the benefits to all his colleagues. "I first discovered Alka-Seltzer in high school to relieve stomachaches," he says. "In college a friend taught me to stand on my head to do the same. Over the years I perfected the routine. Now I don't need either. There's no pain."

The role of a student has always appealed to me. Now it feels like an adventure full of possibility.

Back at the health food store, business has picked up with the addition of a brand-new juice bar. Start off easy, carrot with a touch of apple. Then add some greens: cucumbers, watercress, lettuce. All raw, all fresh and, whenever possible, organic.

Even my stint waitressing in a health food restaurant

during my theater days didn't take me this far. Most of my coworkers there believed in the food they served. I remember Doug, the deli man, pledging to drink an eight-ounce cup of carrot juice every day for the rest of his life. "It keeps you young," he grinned, lovingly patting his full head of hair.

This crisis has mobilized me into fighting for my health. I buy three paperbacks on juicing and look for anything that has to do with pregnancy, fertility or cleansing. All of them emphasize the healing effects of green leafy vegetables and the reparative effect of a multitude of nutrients. Since the food is already liquid, it's easily assimilated and used by the body. This I like.

We buy a small vegetable juicer at Zabar's. Ellena is almost two years old and eminently capable of making all the key decisions in our morning juicing ritual. She stands on one of the kitchen chairs and reaches into the bowl of freshly cut vegetables. "Do we stay with carrots?" I ask. "Go for a deeper orange?"

She nods.

"How would a piece of apple affect the color? Add more lettuce and parsley?"

"Red, red!" she yells. Two slices of beet slide into the chute, and within seconds the counter is covered with red fingerprints. After she blends the perfect hue, she puts in a straw and empties the glass.

The change in our eating habits liberates Ellena from food assault. I no longer follow her around with bits of food, sneaking something in each time she opens her mouth. She eats everything I do and drinks a glass of fresh juice a day. I know she is getting enough nutrients.

On one of my pilgrimages to the health food store, I see a rugged-looking young man gulp down a one-ounce shot of green liquid with a satisfied air. "Boy, this stuff really cleans you out," he says. What? I innocently ask for an ounce. The smell hits me first and causes my stomach to tighten in dreaded anticipation. I decide to down it in one shot, which turns out to be a mistake. The nausea shoots up as I fight my gag reflex. I pour some carrot juice down my throat in an attempt to mask the taste. Ugh, I can't do this.

Yet, I'm intrigued, especially when I see a number of articles and an entire book dedicated to the healing effects of drinking it. Wheatgrass is, well, grass. It is alive, delivered to health food stores and juice bars in trays of soil, juiced with a special press that squeezes out the liquid. The stuff is sold by the ounce. One shouldn't overindulge too quickly. Ann Wigmore, the author of *Wheatgrass Juice,* and the foremost advocate of the medicinal use of wheatgrass in America, talks about wheatgrass chlorophyll, extracted from seven-day-old wheat sprouts, as a powerful invigorator and an overall tonic. It's too bad my stomach tightens up just thinking about it.

One night, just as I'm ready to turn off the light, check in on Ellena, and quietly slip into bed, a paragraph in *The Juicing Book* by Stephen Blauer leaps from the page directly into my ovaries. It talks about a study in which two months on wheatgrass juice reversed infertility in cows. The next morning I'm at the juice bar before Theresa takes the CLOSED sign off the register. "*Czesc,* Ellenka," she says warmly, then gives me a look of alarm when I order an ounce of the hard stuff. I get a cup of filtered water to use as a chaser, take a deep breath, and start drinking. The taste and smell have become irrelevant. I line up my shot glass and water every morning, the way my mother used to line up my daily dose of cod liver oil.

Wanting a baby provides incentives to eat or drink anything that promises to improve my odds. Just the fact that I've been able to pull it off, to transform in a relatively short time from a mere mortal requiring an afternoon coffee and chocolate cake into a tempeh enthusiast, is a giant boost for my bruised self-esteem. It helps me see myself as more fluid, alterable.

More important, moving forward helps me climb out of the feeling of defeat. That, right now, is as strong a motivator as the need to get pregnant. I am pouring all my frustration and pain into action. If I don't conceive, at least I'll have the healthiest body I've ever had.

7

FISHING WITH
THE YOGIS

*. . . that with the exercise of self-trust,
new powers shall appear.*

—RALPH WALDO EMERSON

While Ellena takes her nap, I sit at the kitchen counter going over my students' journal entries. I've taken two of my classes from Hunter to a small theater in Greenwich Village to see *The Fantasticks,* billed as "the longest-running musical in the world." We've spent two weeks reading the play and listening to the music, and I'm inspired to see that the work has paid off.

"Most of all we can see the actors very closely and sometimes I felt as if I am actor. And the pianist played with putting her all emotion into play. She was closing her eyes and shaking her head and I fell in the music perfectly," writes Sho from Japan.

Jaisuk wants to see the show again with his wife who arrives from Korea next week. "I cannot forget Sullivan St. Playhouse forever ever. Because we have read the script already I noticed I could catch the words and that is great experience for me."

It's almost three o'clock. The nurse from the IVF clinic should be calling back with the results of this month's FSH. I've been a vegetarian for four months, my sinus headaches are history, and my expectations are rising, though, so far, my FSH hasn't dropped below 34.

The call arrives. 29! Thirteen points lower than the original 42. It's still too high to change the prognosis, but it feels as if someone pinned a red ribbon of merit on my blouse. The little strip of plastic my first grade teacher awarded to the three best readers in the class, Viera Stefanovicova, Dusan Schmidt, and me.

I want to do more. Like Luisa in *The Fantasticks* I'm ready to "study cloud formations" and "memorize the moon."

For the past few months, Karen has been talking about a new yoga class at the 92nd Street Y.

Over the years I've sampled the various Manhattan yoga studios searching for relief from my lower back pain. Sometimes my teachers would share stories of people who had overcome physical impairments by a systematic practice of specific postures. Why not a hormonal imbalance?

"Doesn't it make sense? Isn't yoga supposed to fix things?" I ask Karen, looking for encouragement. "You should call my teacher, Michael Gilbert. He teaches Iyengar yoga. It's different from anything else I've done. It might be worth having a private class with him," she says, writing down his phone number.

"I haven't worked with anyone with your particular problem before," says Michael when I call. "But I can show you a few postures that are beneficial for the reproductive organs."

In a small study in his Upper East Side apartment, he takes me through a series of postures. "We'll start with a couple of standing poses. Initially you can do them supported against the wall, so that you won't get exhausted by them. They will generally strengthen your system." He places a small wooden block next to my foot in case my arm doesn't quite reach the floor.

"Just by standing up straight, you lengthen the spine and give more room to the abdominal organs and the ovaries because they're no longer compressed. You're also working the muscles around the uterus so that they become firm and more vital," he says quietly. "Now let the shoulders release. What you're doing is creating an inner lift. That's the other thing about yoga. It works on the inner organs in addition to strengthening the skeletal body. The lungs are lifting, the diaphragm is lifting. Now bring your arms up. Stretch them all the way. A little more. Draw the muscles of the upper arms into the elbows. Suck them in. That's it. Good work."

I have done some of the poses before, but this calls for much more concentration. Michael keeps speaking: "Pull your kneecaps up so you get your hamstrings lengthened. Now lengthen the inner arms. Get into the stretch."

My head is spinning. "The only parts of the feet that are lifted are the toes. The mounds of the toes grip the floor." I'm going to have to take a course in anatomy. What is that song they sing on *Sesame Street?* The shin bone's connected to the knee bone, the knee bone's connected to the . . .

As if he were eavesdropping on my thoughts, Michael's voice chimes in: "The brain doesn't get caught up in the struggle. The brain is an observer."

Next, he helps me get into a shoulder stand. But my leg and stomach muscles are too weak to hold the position. Michael places a couple of blankets on the floor next to a folding chair, another blanket on the seat. Once in the pose, my legs rest against the back of the chair. This way, I can hold the position much longer and heighten its healing effect.

On the way out Michael hands me a list of instructors on the West Side: "You might try a couple of these teachers. Robin Janis is wonderful. And she is somewhere in your neighborhood." He's sending me to a competitor. I guess that's the Zen approach to building up your clientele.

"If nothing else, making my body stronger can only help," I tell myself on the way to the crosstown bus. I feel energized by the workout and taking action. Have I just treated myself to a private class? One whole teacher all to myself? What blasphemous self-indulgence. A slight detour from the skimping, self-sacrificing approach I usually apply to getting through the day. I feel like a well-fed kid in a brand-new winter jacket. I might as well face it. I want to be taken care of. No, not just taken care of. I want to be pampered.

"The good of the collective comes before your own. Only the decadent bourgeois put their own interests before those of the people." Those were the socialist slogans of my youth mirrored in every school poster. But self-denial doesn't work for me anymore.

A week after my private session, I try a class with Robin Janis. I'm fifteen minutes early, but the small studio is already busy with a dozen people chatting and stretching as they wait for the class to begin. Lined up against the wall are neat stacks of colorful Mexican blankets (the colors alone could send an egg into a mad dash up the fallopian tube), light blue sticky mats, a basket of white cotton belts, and a row of wooden blocks.

"Is there anything special you want to work on?" Robin asks.

"I'm trying to get pregnant," I reply, as she smoothes out the blanket under my shoulders.

"Congratulations," she says. She must have misunderstood, I say to myself.

"Congratulations on trying to get pregnant," she adds matter-of-factly.

Robin is not much taller than five four, but her firm muscles exude strength well beyond her size. Standing in the middle of the room in her wine-colored shorts and matching tank top, her abundant wavy brown hair loosely covering her shoulders, she is the best advertisement for yoga practice. A master of what one of my professors in graduate school called "teaching on your feet," Robin addresses whatever questions come up.

She calls us over to check Mary's headstand. "Are her arms parallel? Which arm does she need to bring in? Her arms must be parallel, otherwise she has no stability." The instruction is highly individual. She is familiar with each student's idiosyncrasies: "See, watch. Hailey tends to over-extend her shoulders. That creates tension in her upper back."

We learn from each other as we watch her adjust some-one's posture, lifting this and that, turning a knee inward, tucking a pelvic bone under. Every time we accomplish an *asana,* posture, there is something new to work on. Robin takes us through each pose as if we were looking at it through a magnifying glass, isolating each movement, then the next and the next, until the last stretch. Then holding it a little longer to give the body a chance to reap the ben-efits. Then letting go.

Once again, ribs, joints; all those bones I have to get reacquainted with. It's embarrassing how little I know about the workings of my body.

"Put the belts around your upper arms. That way you don't have to think about keeping them in place," says our teacher, walking around the room. "Is this legal?" groans a bearded man in his fifties as Robin pulls the belt a little tighter to keep his arms in alignment.

The use of props like small wooden blocks, rods, belts, and chairs is important in the Iyengar method. They help a weak muscle to stay in the pose, or compensate for partic-ular idiosyncrasies of each body. Knowing when and how to use a particular prop is an art in itself.

"The more precise the poses, the more profound their effect on the body," says Robin, as we carefully arrange fin-gers and spread toes.

I feel as if all this tightening of muscles slowly lifts my spirits as much as my ribs. Each *asana* is a bugle call for all the parts of my body to join in the battle. It's hard to feel helpless doing the "warrior" with your arms extended, chest lifted, thighs hardened.

Robin tells me about a special Friday morning class for pregnant women. "Bobby Clennell is teaching it right now. She knows a great deal about women's issues. She'll be a wonderful person for you to talk to."

The parquet floor of the studio at the Iyengar Institute on Twenty-fourth Street is sprinkled with small and not-so-small pouches and bellies in various stages of bloom. Some look like any minute now a little head is going to burst through like an oversized belly button.

I'm late. The class must have started a few minutes ago. I'm prepared to tell Bobby I'm late because of the inconsiderate people on the subway, how at least three times during my ride, the conductor had to ask people to step away from the door. But before I could take a breath, Bobby walks over to me with a blanket and a belt. She helps me get the belt around my upper arms. In the next few minutes she says something I should write in red crayon and tape on my refrigerator: "Yoga is probably the only exercise, if you can call it that, which actually targets the hormonal system. The upside down poses are very important because they stimulate the connection between the ovaries and the pituitary gland." The momentum of that sentence alone will keep me going for several months.

More treats appear on the way: "This next pose is the best invention for women," says Bobby, taking us through a variation of the triangle pose. "It stretches the abdomen, creates lots of space inside you, lots of space for your inner organs. Also, when you release the shoulder and open up the chest, the heart center opens. You become emotionally more stable and that also affects your hormone levels."

At this point, I'm beginning to wonder if someone has tipped her off, let her know I was coming. Maybe one of my friends told her I was desperate to get pregnant and that hearing something positive could make a real difference.

Her voice is as soft as a blanket of snowflakes. "You're sending a message into your nervous system, your endocrine system, telling it, okay, now you can work. I've taken some of the pressure off you. Here's a little help. Now you can do what you're supposed to do."

My unconscious hears: *You came to the right place. Stick around.*

At some point toward the end of the class, she comes over to me with more blankets: "I want you to be able to relax your legs," she says. Then she gently lowers my chin. "If the chin is up, the head is noisy. That's it." My body softens, lets go.

For a few minutes, someone else is in charge. There is nothing for me to take care of. No last-minute instructions for the sitter as I peel Ellena's hands off my shoulders and

84 hand her over. No poking my head through the door with just one more detail: "Could you put some moisturizer on her legs? They're very dry. Oh, and you need to steam the carrots a little longer, the last time they were too hard." Then a quick run for the subway.

Tears of gratitude roll down my cheeks. Gratitude for finding a place to do what I'm doing. For the luxury of being able to lie here, for the sturdy support of the folded blanket underneath my lower back. The comfort emanating from the dozen or so bodies in the spacious sun-filled studio.

I open my eyes. On the wall directly in front of me is a photograph of Iyengar. He is balanced on his left leg, his left arm is extended in front of him, the right arm is lifted and bent behind his back touching the sole of his right foot. Looking at him, I can sense the absolute, stubborn commitment of his body. It feeds my faith.

Bobby's voice guides me back to myself. "Draw your attention inward. Mother Earth is calling you to relax. Relax your jaw. Rest the thumb. If the thumb is active, the brain is active. Let your body receive rather than give." The sound of those words reminds me why I came here. Having a baby is giving, giving, and more giving. Maybe I just need to take for a while before I start a new round of giving.

Moments later, I look around, taking in the sleepy surrender of the other women's bodies scattered across the parquet floor. A stage of dancers at rest. Then, on cue, a choreography of bodies slowly turning, torsos lifting, one at a time. "The head comes up last." Bobby's voice brings us back into the room. The class is over. For me, the work has just begun.

During my first year in America, a time when I had felt disconnected from everyone, including myself, my cousin Lillian would occasionally invite me to spend a weekend with her family. Their home was filled with warmth. Her husband, Miles, served her breakfast in bed on Sunday mornings, a thoughtfully arranged tray with a single rose in a tiny glass bottle. It was a place where people listened with interest when someone spoke and asked questions that showed they understood what the other person said.

After a weekend at Lillian's, I would go back to New Jersey feeling that as long as I could once in a while fill up on a chunk of their love, I would be okay.

The studio on Twenty-fourth Street feels like such an oasis.

It's reassuring to be touched by Bobby as she adjusts my posture. It makes me realize how often I wish I were less self-conscious about hugs and touching and more physical with my women friends.

I try to attend the Friday morning class as much as I can. Seeing all those bellies reminds my body that we're all made of the same stuff, and that the possibility of having what they have is within me. It's a place where I can connect with people who believe that what they are doing profoundly changes them. Such places and such people help me strengthen the voice that tells me to trust my own judgment. The voice that gives me the authority to decide what does and does not make sense.

86   I feel as if my body and I are starting over. Our *guruji,* which is the way insiders refer to Iyengar, has opened up a brand-new world for us. On the surface, I seem to be in reasonably good shape. I'm five feet one and three quarters of an inch tall and weigh a hundred and seven pounds. Not too much fat or flailing flesh. I diligently go through the Nautilus circuit at the gym, ride my stationary bike at least three times a week, and follow the Chinese doctor's advice to jump rope.

Yet there is so much swept under the rug. Oceans of tension, weak muscles, shallow breathing, no real attention paid to this much-used piece of equipment that is meant to stay in good working order for a lifetime.

Experimenting with the postures at home is a little like learning a new language. I can do a pose a hundred times, each time increasing my fluency. And my yoga language is getting richer, more detailed. I'm learning how to tune in to signals, listen to what my body is trying to tell me. Most days, it says: "Hang in there. If there is something you want, hold on to it. I'll get to it as soon as I'm ready. Right now I need lots of room. Room to let go, stretch, breathe. Time to slowly fill up with air."

Throughout my life I have been engaged in two kinds of magical thinking. One, a belief that there is some other-worldly force outside myself, a Goddess of restitution, who will one day reach out a willowy hand and pull me from the wings onto center stage. There will be cheering and applause, and all the worldly riches that up to now have eluded me will be hung around my neck.

The other is a more authentic kind of magic. In the course of my life, I had periodically caught sight of it through curtains of depression, yet until now, whenever I reached out my hand to touch it, it slipped away. The magic I'm talking about is the realization that something you believe to be impossible is, in fact, possible. That in spite of what anyone has ever told you, your fate is not sealed.

Doing my daily yoga practice brings this realization closer. There are still days when I open my hand and find that it's empty. I get tired of cheering myself on. "You're a fool," the old voice says. "You sure know how to make things up. Why don't you just give thanks for what you have and obsess about something else." Then I see my red yoga blanket at the bottom of the closet, and I realize that I can't turn back. The current's got me. All I can do is keep rowing and see where it takes me.

There is a difference between having an idea that yoga is good for my body and noticing my hands don't tremble as much in the handstand; or feeling the tension slowly leave my body at the end of the day as I do my simple but amazingly effective forward bend. All I do is stand about a foot away from the wall and bend forward. My buttocks touch the wall. With each exhalation I let the weight of my arms and torso pull me a little more toward the floor.

Turned upside down in a shoulder stand, my toes reaching up toward the ceiling, I believe I can turn things around. Whatever my FSH tells me, I can turn it on its head.

The upside-down poses appeal to Ellena as well. On

88 Sunday mornings, she lies between Ed and me, kicking her legs up into a shoulder stand. She squeals in delight as Ed holds her by the ankles and moves her legs back and forth, yelling, "No walking on the ceiling."

The work brings an awareness to the most remote, least-known parts of my body. Like little points of light in a World War II movie I once saw. The voice of the narrator jubilantly announced the names of all the cities liberated by the Soviets. With each name, another light on the map blinked. Similarly, I envision squadrons of cells blinking awake on the map of my body.

Late at night, I spread my blanket over the bathroom tiles and lie with my arms spread at my side, palms up. My back is slightly arched and supported by a bolster. I'm wide open.

Suddenly my body remembers lying just like this. In my mind's eye I see my obstetrician standing at the foot of the labor bed, screaming, "Anesthesia, I need anesthesia now. I have to get this baby out now." She turns to me as arms reach out pushing the stretcher into the operating room. "I'm sorry we don't have time for an epidural, we have to put you under," she says.

I nod, trying to stay calm. I mustn't let my terror seep through to the baby. "Just take deep breaths," says Ed, holding my hand. But he looks scared.

In the operating room, my doctor pleads with the anesthesiologist: "Can I cut? Can I cut now? Let me know when I can cut." Then from somewhere very far away, across the expanse of my burning belly, I hear the loud moaning of my own voice. A white shadow bends over me: "Ms. Indichova, you have a healthy daughter."

My body hasn't forgotten Ellena's birth. It doesn't have to be this scary next time.

The meditative nature of yoga helps me heal. "The eye of the soul is just a little above the space between your brows. If that is still, your soul is still," says Bobby in one of her classes.

The soul? It was a forbidden word throughout my childhood. Spirituality in the Czechoslovak Socialist Republic was synonymous with religion, and religion meant being against the Party. Party members had no religion. Even if you were just an ordinary citizen, it was better if you were not seen anywhere near a church or a synagogue.

My parents drew strength from their Jewish heritage, but God and the existence of the soul were not widely discussed at our dinner table. Spirituality was connected with sadness, as if my parents, who were Holocaust survivors, had been let down by their faith, and they didn't want us to rely on ours too much.

As a child, lying in bed at night, I silently recited the short prayer my parents taught us: "Dear God, my eyes are closing now, but may yours be watching over me while I sleep, and watching over my parents and my dear sister so that with the morning sun we can embrace each other again." Then I went through a short ritual, which consisted of a series of images, such as my mother bending over me and stroking my hair or my sister helping me with my penmanship. These images were to purge me of any less than pure feelings I might have felt for them on a particular day. If I fought a lot with my sister that day, I would try to come up with extra footage of her performing good deeds.

As an adult, I've always felt vaguely embarrassed about my need for some form of spiritual practice. Such things didn't seem a very productive use of my time. At the same time I yearned for a place and a time to surrender. To take my hands off the control panel and trust that someone else will keep things going. That my child will keep breathing and that Ed will come home from work and no one will drop anything on our heads.

Doing my yoga practice, I'm learning that I can't afford not to feed my soul. Not if I want to be able to get up each morning and move forward with my work.

A wise, peaceful seer inside me tells me that all is well, my baby is on its way. I do my *asana*s to strengthen her voice as I used to do scales to strengthen my singing voice. With every shoulder stand, I give my intuition a standing ovation for hanging in there, even when she's told to turn her back on me.

At times I even feel that what I'm going through is a good thing. My unborn child is teaching me how to slow down and pay attention, and how to be nicer to myself.

On other days a dull ache reminds me how badly I want to get pregnant. The possibility that I may not be able to still hurts. To do all that I'm doing and accept the fact that I may not get pregnant again would be a good place to work from. But can I ever get there?

I am, I realize, the perennial student. One day in graduate school, we talked about how to give our students a sense of autonomy and how to teach them to correct their own writing and to hear their own mistakes. At the beginning of the discussion, the professor wrote on the blackboard: "Give a man a fish and you will feed him for a day. Teach him how to fish and you will feed him for a lifetime."

The more I practice, the more I understand that this work is profoundly changing me. Everything I do—the exactness of the poses, the depth of the breath, the commitment to the precision of each pose—is transforming my vision of what is possible.

8

SPRING
CLEANING

Now I scan the New Age magazines for life-enhancing formulas the way some people check for the hottest stock to add to their portfolios. Since most of these publications are issued monthly or bimonthly, I often end up thumbing through the same issue for several weeks. Each magazine has a classified section where health professionals describe their services. There are almost no direct references to treating infertility, but many of the regimens promise to revitalize one's body, mind, and soul.

Today, as I skim through the pages, the word "rejuvenation," printed in bold letters, draws my attention to an ad for internal cleansing. Reading through it, I'm reminded of a scene in *L.A. Story,* where Sarah Jessica Parker, the ultimate New Age seductress, tells a depressed Steve Martin that a high colonic could give him a new start. When I first saw the movie, I thought she was talking about some exotic drink. What she meant, as Steve correctly guessed, was a fancy enema.

My body has been giving me lots of red ribbons for my new eating habits. Last week, Ed remarked that he hasn't heard me complain about my rheumatism, which had been part of my life since college. Often, the pain in my legs would get me out of bed in the middle of the night in search of Extra Strength Tylenol. I had completely forgotten about all that.

The overzealous student in me wants to show I can do even better. Maybe a colonic could push me yet a few more inches forward.

I call one of the ads. "If you would like an overview of colonic irrigation and its potential benefits, press one," says the computerized voice. The crash course that follows tells me that this form of internal cleansing was practiced in ancient Egypt and is a part of many healing regimens. "Proper elimination is one of the most important processes essential to good health," the recording continues. "Material deposits build up along the colon wall and cause nutritional deficiencies no matter how good your diet is. Our experience proves beyond doubt that poor colon management lowers the body's resistance and predisposes it to many degenerative and chronic diseases." The voice ends with a spunky "The cleaner you are within, the cleaner you are without."

Among the benefits mentioned are improved circulation, increased energy, elimination of allergies, and better skin tone. Infertility is not on the list, but if all goes well, the energy boost will spill over into my ovaries.

94   By now a seasoned consumer of alternative modalities, I
have become more cautious in my choice of practitioners.
One ad's phone is answered by a woman with a French accent. When I tell her I'd like to come by and meet her first,
she is quite accommodating. "You can come any day. Just
make sure you are here about ten minutes before the hour.
I'll be happy to show you around."

Patti, a petite blonde with a warm smile, greets me at the
door. Everything in the office, including Patti, is spotless.
She takes me for a quick tour into the small treatment room
with a narrow massage table covered with a white sheet.

"We use a gravitational method," says Patti, pointing to a
large tank of water above the table. "The water flows from
an elevated tank downward. There are two tubes attached to
a speculum. One tube brings the water into your body and
the other one directs it into the sewage system." When I ask
her if the process is painful, she says: "If you are bloated it
can be a little uncomfortable, but I wouldn't say it's painful."

I like Patti, but for the sake of comparison I decide to
visit one of the health centers in Greenwich Village. Along
the walls of the large waiting room are glass cases filled with
books and supplements. Men and women in white lab coats
appear, then disappear behind a drawn curtain. Beyond it
are several treatment rooms. In a small alcove next to
the receptionist, two elegantly dressed women with head-
phones are watching an instructional video with diagrams
of the digestive system. The waiting room is busy, and no
one seems to question my presence.

I walk over to a bulletin board covered with ads for wa-

ter filters, air filters, and machines that ionize the air and replace ozone. In the corner I notice a light green leaflet with
a fable: "When God made man, the various parts of the
body argued which part was the boss. The brain said, 'I am.
I send all the signals.' The hands said they were, as they
could make him anything he wanted. The feet said they
were, as they could take him anywhere. They all claimed to
be most important. The colon listened quietly and said to
himself, 'I'll show you who is the boss.' He clogged up. The
feet could not carry him, the hands fell limp, the heart was
ready to stop pumping and everything got jammed up."

This office is definitely quite legitimate and a lot more
high-tech than Patti's one-woman operation. Still, I feel
more comfortable with her.

This time I get to settle into the comfortable sofa in
Patti's waiting room with a cup of tea and a long question-
naire about my medical history, diet, and health concerns.
When I tell Patti the reason for my visit she seems genuinely interested in helping me. "I'm not a certified nutri-
tionist, so officially I should not be recommending herbs,
but have you tried raspberry tea? It's meant to strengthen
the uterus. Oatstraw is also good for any uterine problems."
She hands me a folded gown and adds, "Getting your body
as clean as possible is a great idea."

A few minutes later we are both at our stations. All systems are go. Patti reassures me: "I will stay with you during the entire treatment. In a minute you will start filling
up with water. Let me know when you feel full. Otherwise
there is nothing you have to do. Just relax and let it hap-

pen. If you feel any discomfort, let me know. We can always stop." As she speaks she is gently pressing on acupressure points along my shin.

One side of my abdomen starts to cramp. Patti massages the spot. Her touch and presence are soothing. Any minute now she could get up and make me some tea and toast and read me a story. Her chatter takes my attention away from the tumultuous activities in my belly.

"One of my clients brought me an article about all these famous people who used to get colonics, like Mae West and Gloria Swanson. Supposedly Princess Di had one every Thursday. So you are in good company." We have a good forty-five minutes ahead of us. It gives us plenty of time for a woman-to-woman exchange, which leads to a discussion of the opposite sex. Patti, who is thirty-three, is much encouraged to hear that I got married at thirty-nine and even happier to learn that Ed is almost seven years younger than I am.

"That's great. It makes me feel like there is still hope. I have just been meeting the wrong men lately. They are either married, or they just got divorced and want to date sixteen-year-olds, or they are just weird," she says.

"What does your husband do? He used to be a chef? So he cooks for you. You're so lucky."

From time to time she comments on the effectiveness of the treatment. "You are getting rid of a lot of stuff you don't need. I just know this will make a difference," she says. "After all, the ovaries are not far from the organs of elimination, so it makes perfect sense to keep the area in the best possible shape."

My time is almost up. The cramping has stopped, but I'm feeling a little tired. In a few minutes Patti helps me off the table and points me toward the adjacent bathroom.

A light-headed exhaustion spreads through my body, the kind one feels after a long day at the beach. I hope I can stay awake until I get home.

Patti urges me to chew my food more, drink more water, to make sure I have at least one large salad a day, and to take a supplement of acidophilus. "It would be great for you to do a raw juice fast one day every couple of weeks," she says. She hands me a folder with some reading material and off I go.

Over the next few days my eyes seem less tired, and my skin is clearer.

I follow Patti's advice to eat more salads, try to eat more slowly, and remind myself to drink more water. My first raw juice fast is easier than I thought.

I drop hints to several of my friends about the wonders of getting unclogged. Most of them look at me as if I am talking about a new hallucinogenic. At best, they say it's not the kind of thing they could ever subject themselves to. Still, with all the bad press among my friends and the general controversy about the invasiveness of colonic treatment, all I can say is, I went, I saw, and I conquered what could have been enemies to my well-being. My body is like a house after a spring cleaning, with the furniture moved around, the floors scoured, every inch of surface wiped clean. A safe place for a baby.

9

An Inside Job

> To begin to live in the present we must first make
> amends with our past, . . . and we can do it only by . . .
> extraordinary, unceasing labor.
>
> —ANTON CHEKHOV, *The Cherry Orchard*

My ovaries ache and I take a cab to see my gynecologist. She says I have a cancerous tumor in my uterus. It is a punishment for wanting another baby. Dozens of arms lift me onto a stretcher and wheel me into the operating room. Several doctors in surgical masks walk in and take turns bending over me, pressing on my abdomen. "As soon as you stop trying to get pregnant again, we'll help you with the tumor," says one. Then he signals the others to file silently out of the room.

I wake up with a start, my hand unconsciously rubbing my belly. The panic subsides as I see Ed. The bedroom door is half open and I look toward Ellena asleep in her crib in the corner of the living room.

I have been focusing on my body. Eating green and yel-

low foods, doing *asanas*. I've seen the results almost immediately. But changing the way I think and feel is more
daunting, at best slow and tedious.

I forgot about the most important body part. The invisible CEO that sits in the corner office of my head, gener-
ating all the important memos. She's not letting me get
away with it.

A familiar voice of warning is making its way to the surface: "Better halt while you're ahead, count your blessings,
and stop clamoring for more."

Oh no. Not again. After all the years of analysis, meditation, chanting, and consciousness-raising workshops, you
would think I was done with the need to punish myself. To
keep paying for the privilege of being alive.

I was born in 1949 in Kosice, Czechoslovakia, a small
city near the Hungarian border. Four years earlier, my
mother, Edita, returned from Auschwitz, a concentration
camp in Poland. My father had been liberated from a camp
in Germany called Matthausen. My two grandmothers, my
father's sister Adele, my mother's first husband and her
eight-year-old son, Robert, were murdered by the Nazis.

Four years is not a very long time. It wasn't long enough
to stop my parents' grieving. So their sorrows became our
sorrows.

"Matthausen was a big place," my father told us. "It
looked like a giant tent. Outside, the dead were piled up
high. Inside, we slept close together in rows. Some of us
worked in mines, and others stacked up corpses. We got a
little bit of water and a tiny piece of bread you could swal-

low in one mouthful. I was in bad shape; the one thought that kept me going was—what would my mother say if I didn't come home—but there were also days when I no longer cared about what happened to me."

After the war my father returned to his hometown. "I went to the house we lived in before deportation. Someone else was living in our small apartment. The neighbor gave me a winter coat and a small ring, with a note, "Children, love each other. You will not see me again.""

He later found out that his mother died in the cattle car on the way to the camps. She was fifty-four years old. My father's younger sister and her husband were murdered six months before the end of the war.

My sister, Susan, and I soaked up images of my mother's daily life in the camp until they were as much a part of our emotional life as if we had lived them.

"The dust everywhere was suffocating. We slept in low, wooden huts with beaten earth floors. Instead of bunks there were bare planks; up to nine of us slept on each plank—when you turned in the middle of the night you woke up everybody else. From the tiny window I could see flames of the cremation furnace.

"Periodically we had to line up naked, for head count. Making eye contact with the guards could cost you your life. They would just point to someone and that was it. Maybe they didn't like the way she held her head or the expression on her face. The best thing was to make yourself invisible."

My half-brother Robert, whom everyone came to

know as Robika, the red-haired little boy whose face looked out at us from photographs throughout our house, was a very real member of our family. In one snapshot he is three years old, dressed in checkered tailored shorts with suspenders, a matching jacket, his hat askew revealing a wisp of hair. He is standing against a field of daisies—eyes full of mischief and expectation—as if he is about to divulge some terrific secret.

Sitting by our bed in the evening, my mother sang, *"Tente, babam, tente.* Hush, baby, hush." It was the same lullaby she used to sing to him, she told us. She kept her son alive by retelling countless stories of his short life. "One day I sent him to the corner store to buy eggs. On his way home he saw a chimney sweep across the street. Now, you know, when you see a chimney sweep you have to grab your button for good luck. So he grabbed his button with both hands and the eggs turned into a yellow puddle in the middle of the sidewalk." My mother smiled at the memory.

There were other ways to make sure we didn't forget him. Whenever we were on vacation, if we happened to see a young man with red hair who was the same age Robika would have been had he survived, one of us posed the question: "Do you think it's him? Should we ask his name?" Of course, we all knew Robika could not be alive. Yet I had never stopped yearning for his return and had secretly invented dozens of ways for his escape, and each time we approached one of these strangers, I held my breath. Part of me believed that one day we would find him. One day he'd be back, and we would all be one happy family.

102   My parents loved us and took great pleasure from their "little pearls," the name my mother coined for Susan and me. Yet beneath their cheerful faces was darkness. It was like the thirteenth room in the enchanted castle that no one was allowed to enter. Sometimes I tried to imagine the secrets hidden there.

I thought about the morning of deportation. The anguish my mother must've felt as she packed her small son's belongings for the journey. What did she tell him? How did she comfort him? How did she comfort herself? How did she say good-bye? In my mind's eye I saw Robika walking off with his father while my mother lined up with the women. But I never asked for any of these details. The stories my parents didn't tell us, the ones they didn't dare think about remained locked in that forbidden room.

Still, the feelings of guilt and self-blame were telegraphed through my father's chronic uncontrollable fits of rage, my mother's lack of care in her appearance, the chaos and the absence of objects other than the essentials, in our home. No objects of beauty. That would have been a sign of indulgence, or arrogance, implying they had forgotten the past.

Now look at all I have. A beautiful, healthy child, a great husband, a wonderful life in America. How dare I ask for more? No matter how much my rational self assures me that I have the right to be happy, I can't stop looking over my shoulder, wondering what apocalypse is hurtling toward me. I'm always ready to sacrifice, to pack up, to capitulate. To abdicate to someone else who knows better.

When I emigrated to America at nineteen, those who "knew better" convinced me that my age and accent made me unable to continue the career in the theater that I had started when I was eight. Acting had always been my reliable source of joy. Nothing could touch me onstage. The taunting of my peers vanished. It was like telling everyone: "Go ahead, search me if you need to. You'll find nothing. Go on, open the cupboards. You'll find no crime to charge me with." Yet when my advisers spoke of the futility of an artistic career, I stopped for the next ten years, without offering much resistance. I wanted to prove I could sacrifice and be good like my parents. "Don't ask for more. Bury your longing and never ask for anything more." That's what the rational voices of wisdom had told me.

Maybe that's what this is all about. Maybe that's why I can't give up now. I gave up too many times before.

As my favorite cousin Lillian often reminds me, in Chinese the symbol for crisis is the same as the symbol for opportunity. Becoming a member of the infertility subculture breathes new life into old skeletons.

My infertility tells me something's wrong with me. But then, there has always been something wrong with me. Suddenly, I'm back in seventh grade, longing to be just like the mohair-sweatered girls who talked about kissing boys and walked over to each other's houses to investigate hairstyles. I wanted to be one of them instead of the *Zhidovka*, Jew Girl. The word was synonymous with a curse or a shameful disease. Everyone knew I was a carrier.

What I need now is a crash course in self-acceptance, in

deserving happiness rather than being threatened by it. A voice strong enough to silence the echoes of the past.

My first teacher shows up during a trip with my sister and her family. My brother-in-law, who is in perpetual search for enlightenment, is listening to a "You can do it if you really want to" tape in the car. In the past I would have exchanged a knowing look with my sister and dozed off. Today I need a miracle, and Dr. Wayne Dyer tells me I could make magic.

I buy several of his books that assure the reader anything is possible. Every night I sit on our cozy tiled bathroom floor getting my pep talk from Dr. Dyer. I feel foolish reading him over and over, but I'm hungry for what he says. It isn't a crime to be happy. Being happy does not insult the dead. I need to hear it. I need someone to tell me it's okay for me to get what I want.

Because even though it's been thirty-five years since story time with my parents, the feeling their past left in me seems to be frozen in time. The seven-year-old in me walked away with the feeling that life has its price. Suffering is the payment. I should have saved my parents from the Nazis.

I know the idea is preposterous. How could I have possibly saved them when I wasn't even born? Yet all my life it has been my truth.

It's much easier for me to understand this now that I'm a mother. I recognize the instantaneous transfer of feeling between parent and child through an invisible pipeline. When I'm elated, Ellena laughs along with me. When I'm

rushed, on edge, I see her turn in fear. "Are you angry?"
she asks, thinking she did something wrong. Foolish as it
sounds, it seems I have to forgive myself for crimes I did
not commit. Dr. Dyer, as well as other authors that are beginning to wander into my life, is helping me.

Even my closest friends sometimes waver in their support. They may be afraid to give false hope, or they may be
uncomfortable with the pain. They may have their own list
of setbacks, their own belief in the futility of reaching for
something they want. In some cases there's a wish, however
unconscious, to commiserate rather than rejoice.

Ed has recently started a new job, and after twelve hours
at work, he often sits at his newly installed computer on the
kitchen counter late into the night. I hide my sadness, trying to spare him, knowing it only makes him feel helpless.
He eats tempeh and stands on his head on his yoga blanket
and saves up his sperm until the right time of the month,
but he is also afraid to be too hopeful.

The writers of my guidebooks have nothing at stake.
They're available at a moment's notice twenty-four hours a
day. I open the book and there they are, encouraging, supportive, helpful. The enemies of doubt and despair, they
help me understand my guilt and dispense absolution as
many times as I choose to read the appropriate chapter.

Dr. E, a homeopath, introduces me to another ally and
teacher, Dr. Epstein. "He's been quite successful treating a
wide range of problems through imagery. I think you
would find his book on healing visualizations quite interesting," she says in accented English.

Seeing images in our minds, explains Dr. Epstein in the introduction to his book on visualizations, makes them seem real to you. If you see them often enough, they become real.

He argues that if Western medicine accepts the idea that inducing physiological changes (with antidepressants, for example) can affect the way people feel and think, why is it so difficult to believe the reverse?

I suppose it's true that calling up certain pictures in my mind can bring on instant tears or make me salivate in anticipation. What about my dreams? How often has a sneering face in my dreams sent my heart racing?

What Epstein is telling me is this: By repeatedly calling up images, I am rewiring the circuits of my mind toward a realization of those images.

If this is one tenth as effective as he claims, and if I could, even for a moment, believe it, this would be extraordinary. Yet I have a lifetime of "the right medicine can make it all better" way of thinking to grapple with. The author's picture is on the back cover of the book. Nothing flaky about him. In fact he looks a little like Armin, one of my Eastern European cousins.

When I check the phone book, I see he lives smack in the middle of the Hungarian section. I interpret this as a good omen. I could see if he's for real.

The office is in his apartment; as we meet, I hear the clinking of dishes in the kitchen. I was right, there is something strangely familiar about him. After I present my case, he retrieves a giant medical reference book complete with diagrams. "So let's see, the pituitary which produces the follicle-stimulating hormone is located right here," he says, pointing to the diagram. "The hormone assists in the production of eggs in your ovaries. Your job would be then twofold: to strengthen the ovaries to the point where they wouldn't need such a high level of FSH. And to lower the production of the hormone."

Sitting in his office, bending over charts and reference books, I feel like I'm working with a friend on a particularly challenging homework assignment. "It's very important that you have a clear understanding of the physiology of the problem, the exact location of the organs involved," he says emphatically. He draws an imaginary line between the pituitary and the ovaries, then outlines the journey of the one chosen ripe follicle up through the fallopian tube, where it unites with an eager sperm.

When I'm clear about my mission, I get to sit back, close my eyes, and go for a test drive.

"It's a good idea to do a brief cleansing exercise first," says Dr. Epstein. "Close your eyes, breathe in through your nose and out through your mouth. A nice long exhalation. That's it. Now breathe out three times. See yourself in the middle of a meadow with a flowing stream of crystal-clear water. Take off your clothes and walk into the cool water. There is a small silver bucket on one of the rocks. Use it to pour the water all over your body. As you do this know that you are washing away all the dead cells and impurities from the outside of your body. Now take some water in your cupped hands and drink it. Drink slowly as the water cleans out all the toxins from the inside of your body. Put on a clean robe. Notice its color and texture. And walk out of the meadow. Open your eyes."

No, I'm not exactly having a peak experience, but his words are soothing. "I liked having the whole meadow all to myself. Solitude is a little hard to come by these days," I say. "What kind of sensations should I be looking for? I'm not sure I felt much more than a sense of relaxation."

"That's a good beginning. You may also feel a tingling or heat, sometimes pain or pressure in a particular area of your body. Some images may bring on a powerful emotional reaction. The important thing is, try not to force anything. Let the images come to you. With a little practice and patience your body will become more responsive."

Next we energize my reproductive organs. "Before you begin, tell yourself what it is you want to achieve with this exercise." He takes a handkerchief from his shirt pocket and wipes his forehead.

Again I sit back, close my eyes, turn my attention inward as my guide points out the sights. "See the pituitary gland dispatch the follicle-stimulating hormone. Follow it to the ovaries. First the right one, then the left. How do the ovaries react? What color is the egg? Notice its size." He is there to iron out rough spots, to keep me on track. "Don't linger too much, trying to feel a particular sensation. Just go through it from beginning to end. If you feel the need to do it once more, then go back and start again. Don't make it any longer than you need to. The entire process should take two to three minutes. That doesn't mean you can't be creative and experiment with what works for you. Do it a couple of times a day. The best times are right after you wake up and before you go to bed. Remember, the more specific you can get, the better. Call me if you have any questions. Let me know what happens."

In contrast with many of the fertility specialists I've seen so far, who strived to present me with facts and statistics but shied away from the slightest hint of personal opinion, Dr. Epstein is very direct. "Don't be too quick to put your eggs in a petri dish. Certainly not before you try some alternatives," he says, walking me to the door.

"I couldn't do that even if I wanted to," I reply. "No one would take them. They are supposedly too old."

He smiles and shakes my hand.

Walking up Second Avenue I think how pragmatic Dr. Epstein is, for all his images of meadows and streams. Let's not focus on futility, he seems to be saying.

My daydreaming exercises bring me a rush of freedom. After a while I find that the years of sensory work in my acting classes as well as my lifelong fascination with dreams have been a perfect apprenticeship for imagery. Pictures begin to float in my mind's eye as I experiment with my own exercises. In one of them I'm climbing up a steep mountain. My boots dig into the mud, branches hit my face as I lean against the wind. Suddenly from behind a tree a guide appears offering water, sustenance, a gift for my unborn child. As the climb gets steeper, more and more hands reach out to help. At last a clearing bathed in sunlight reveals a cluster of babies engaged in play. The fragrance of their bodies fills the air as I run to greet them. I decide to call this waking dream The Trail of Faith.

Thus my new daily routine is: healthy food and juices, a chapter from one of my cheerleading books, fifteen minutes of jumping rope, a sequence of yoga postures, and a set of imagery exercises. Over and over, I effortlessly place a switch in my pituitary gland to balance my hormone levels, plant a healthy egg in my uterus, and hike up the trail of faith. I follow this protocol religiously, the way one takes an antibiotic. I wouldn't think of missing a day. Often I don't get more than six hours of sleep, yet I wake up surprisingly rested. If I need to, I can always sneak in a nap with Ellena in the afternoon.

I need to prove to myself that I am serious, and show my body I can be counted on. Tomorrow maybe I'll be more relaxed, more flexible.

But right now, I'm at war. I cannot underestimate the enemy. The most insidious, the most relentless one of them all is the one inside me.

Like a mother of a young child, I take myself by the hand and swing my sword at the monstrous creatures screeching in my head. "Those are only feelings," I tell my-self. I can enlarge them with my timidity or I can ask them to table, offer them a cup of tea, and watch them shrink to human size.

In this struggle I begin to see myself differently, as warriors do. My psyche has been holding out on me.

My parents raised me to be self-defeating, but they also raised me to be strong. They were survivors. In my unwillingness to take no for an answer, I am very much my mother's daughter. When my mother wanted something, she could not be defeated.

In spite of the atrocities she had witnessed, she had a shining faith in the ultimate triumph of good. Her peculiar mixture of agnosticism and faith emerged in the tenet: "God helps those who help themselves." For her it was not a cliché. Exhausted and scarred after her liberation, she was determined to have children again. She knew it was her way back to the living.

Edita was thirty-nine when the war ended, and not a conventional beauty. Her large, protruding teeth overshadowed her blue eyes, her abundant blond hair, and her Roman nose. But she was persistent. The story goes that she plied my father with her special recipe of potatoes and fried onions, got him drunk on homemade buttermilk, seduced him, and, when she became pregnant, gave him the option to leave. She wanted a husband, but a child was a necessity.

Luckily my father, who was five years younger, decided to stay. My mother proceeded against the recommendation of her doctor, who feared that the strain of childbirth on her weakened system would kill her, to have another child. I was that child.

My father has always had an enlightened distrust of authority. A sense that the rules of society were arbitrary, especially if they didn't serve his purposes. In 1974, when getting a visa out of Czechoslovakia was all but impossible, he found a way to get permission for himself and my mother to visit us in America.

He had a reputation in the community for being someone who could get around any problem. His evasions of the
Communist bureaucracy were like little miracles. When
necessities like toilet paper or a loaf of bread were consid-
ered luxury items impossible to find, my father produced
them like a magician. He would tell the right joke to the
right official or buy a drink for a certain "friend." Then
he'd come home holding his prize, howling with laughter
until we all joined in.

I almost forgot the good memories. There were impas-
sioned family poetry readings on Sunday mornings. I never
tired of hearing the one about the boy who stole sausages
from the attic of the old wine-guzzling schoolmaster in the
morning only to give them back to him as gifts in the afternoon. There were backyard ping-pong tournaments,
where I learned to emulate my father's masterful, unreturn-
able slams. There were winters of sledding in the Tatra
mountains and summers of swimming pools in Budapest,
with *palacsintas* (thin pancakes) and hazelnut ice cream.
There are stories and stories to remember. Sooner or later
they'll come back to me. Perhaps someday I can, as Ed's
Grandma Gertie used to say, "Just take the best and leave
the rest."

10

PRESSURE

Hanako, a Japanese woman in my Saturday morning class at Hunter, hands me a pair of origami earrings with two red and gold cranes suspended from a string of white pearls.

"My son school had a celebration last week, I make this for you. Must make a wish," she says, smiling. "They help give you your wish."

Three days later, I get a part of my wish. My FSH is down to 21.4, the lowest it's been since the diagnosis of 42. "If it goes down to at least the mid-twenties, call me." Those were Dr. G's instructions. 21.4 makes me a candidate for drugs.

I leave a message for Dr. G about my new FSH level. A half hour later the doctor calls back with directions: "If you come in this afternoon, the nurse will be showing another couple how to administer the Pergonal shots. Can you and your husband come and join them? You are forty-three years old, and this is the lowest number you've had so far. It may not happen again. Unfortunately, you don't have unlimited time." Her voice sets off the ticking in my head. For a few seconds, I flash through the logistics. I'd have to drop Ellena off with a friend, call Ed. It's almost noon. The appointment is at two. I should be elated.

A few months earlier, before my epiphany at the Health Nuts book section, I might have snapped to attention and obeyed Dr. G's command, but something in me resents the pressure. Like a mare that's being prodded too hard, I want to kick back.

"I'll have to call you back," I say.

Minutes later, I realize I'm not going anywhere. Dr. G tells me to run, my body tells me to slow down. Dr. G says it may not happen again, my body tells me I am getting stronger. Since I have a more intimate relationship with my body than with Dr. G, I choose to listen to the former.

Ed disagrees.

"One of the new guys at work has a cousin who got pregnant on her first cycle of Pergonal. Maybe we should give it a try."

"I just can't do it right now. It feels like a race, and I can't run so fast."

He says he understands.

Nine days later, we double up on production. We are closer than ever before, and just in case there is a sturdy little egg waiting, we'll have a parade of sperm to greet it.

Sometimes during our concentrated baby-making, I

imagine myself extending the tips of my fingers toward otherworldly connections—my mother, who died ten years ago, after fighting off nine progressively more debilitating strokes, and my friend Mark, who died of AIDS five years ago. My mother and Mark, my two allies on the other side. Their ethereal bodies float toward me. If this is a time for heavenly intervention, I know I can count on those two.

My period is a day late. The slightest feeling of dampness sends me running to the bathroom. No, there is no trace of red on the tissue. Not today.

In the morning, the blood comes. The worst part is calling Ed. That's always the first thing I do; the sooner he knows, the sooner he heals. But today I can't seem to remember his work number.

Aside from my worry about Ed, this month is harder than most for me as well. No matter what I told myself, my expectations were high.

For the first time since the diagnosis Ed becomes withdrawn. He is absorbed with Ellena when he comes home and asleep before I get to bed. He leaves for work at the crack of dawn. He barely touches me. I dream I'm a waitress in a restaurant. All the tables are taken. The rest of the staff, the plates, the cutlery, the food, are gone. I'm on my own.

"You think we should have done Pergonal, don't you?" I ask him.

"I'm just tired," he says. His turned back sets off wheels of panic inside me. It brings back the memory of another turned back.

Michael was my first serious relationship. He was tall, a lawyer, and Jewish, and we both knew he was smarter than me. I was working at a dead-end job at ABC. Michael reminded me every day what a low-functioning failure I was. His mission was to emotionally whip me into shape. "We need to talk," he'd say, resting his elbows on the round dining room table. "I'm ambivalent about this relationship. My parents are concerned. They want me to marry someone with an Ivy League education." I sat and cried and wished I were someone his family could approve of. There was more to me than this insecure pleading person. What happened to the other me, the fearless eight-year-old who arranged an audition for herself with a children's theater group and got a job offer on the spot? How could I bring her back?

Michael had the answer. "You were an actress in Czechoslovakia. So act," he said. I accepted the challenge. Getting a part in a play seemed insurmountable. Instead, I put together a one-woman show and performed it in a Manhattan night club to an audience of relatives, acquaintances, and friends. Michael was impressed. I was so elated by his approval and the possibility of performing again that I stopped sleeping and eating, and a week after my American debut I had to check in for a brief vacation at Mount Sinai's psychiatric ward. That was the end of the relationship. An underachiever is one thing, a psychotic underachiever quite another.

Ed is not Michael. I'm not the same person I was twelve years ago.

Today, on my way to a faculty meeting, I catch sight of a familiar figure across the street. It's Ed. He is passing the hardware store, wearing his navy blue suit. He isn't running, but appears to be propelled by an acute need. His body is tilted forward as if to give at least part of him the advantage to get home sooner and make up for all the hours away from his family. All his love for Ellena and me is in that tilt of his walk. I stand there watching him until he turns the corner, then run for the subway.

The pressure is taking a toll on us. What if a year from now we decide we can't wait any longer? "In your case, the only sure thing is adoption," said Dr. C, the first specialist we saw, almost two years ago.

But we do have all that first-grade sperm. If there is a way to pass on a little of Ed to our next baby, it's a chance I can't turn down. By now we have ruled out egg donor IVF. It's too risky, and if we are not successful the first time, the stakes will be so much higher for our next choice. What about surrogacy? The little I know about it comes from following the Mary Beth Whitehead story in the news.

Dr. R, the psychologist at our first specialist's office, gave us the name of a lawyer in Westchester. Charles W and his wife, Connie, help couples find and screen surrogates. His number is still in my notebook.

On the train ride there with Ed I reassure myself that this doesn't mean I have any less faith in my self-prescribed healing regimen. The more options we have, the more relaxed I can be about continuing with my own research.

A woman in her twenties answers the door of a Tudor

suburban house. "I'm Erica, Charles' assistant." She escorts us to a small office off the hallway, points to two easy chairs, and closes the door behind her. On the coffee table in front of us are four massive photo albums. One of them is open. From our vantage point we see snapshots of a smiling brunette sitting on the kitchen floor with a toddler on her knee. Is this a test? Is someone watching us through a two-way mirror? If we reach for the albums, does it mean we're eager enough and therefore pass the admission require-ments? Or if we sit patiently and wait for further instruc-tions, then have we exercised the necessary self-restraint to make us ideal clients?

Ed starts leafing through one of the albums. It's filled with photographs of women. Turning the pages, the faces blend into an assortment of hairstyles and settings, anony-mous smiling faces against the backdrops of kitchens, living rooms, and backyards. Some of the pages include samples of each woman's work, children of all sizes and degrees of cuteness. "I guess this is what we do," says Ed. "Pick some-one we like, then tell the matchmaker, and he'll make all the arrangements."

Charles walks in twenty minutes later apologizing for his lateness. He's a tall, dignified man in his fifties, wearing a beige business suit. Can't quite picture him on the floor chasing a toddler.

Six years ago, Charles and his psychologist wife, after several unsuccessful IVF cycles, hired a surrogate. They have a five-year-old son. "Having been through this our-selves," he says, "we understand the kind of stresses that infertility causes, and we want to do all we can to make this into a joyful experience for you."

"So far the experience has been a little confusing," says Ed with a hint of sarcasm. "It would have been nice to get some sort of an introduction to these albums. We're pretty nervous as it is and to dump us in here for twenty minutes without a word . . ." One more apology and the air is clear enough to proceed.

After we describe our situation, Charles reaches for one of the albums and says, "Why don't we go through these together? If you come across someone you like, I'd be happy to tell you more about her." He turns the pages, commenting. "She is a graduate student who does not expect to have her own children for a while, and she wants to go through a pregnancy before she is thirty. There is a history of breast cancer in her family, and this is her way of trying to beat the odds." The next page shows a couple under a Christmas tree, next to two little girls in identical blue and white polka-dot dresses. Next, a woman with closely cropped hair in her early twenties, pushing a swing. Her small son's mouth is wide open with anticipation.

I feel as if we are house-hunting, following the real estate man through the front door, checking out the square footage, searching for imperfections, commenting: "No, she is much too blond," or "She doesn't look so happy." I'm looking for someone familiar, someone I'd feel an instant bond with, who would have only the best of personality traits to pass on. A spark, a warmth, a soul sister.

"I like her," I say, looking at a picture of a smiling

brunette in jeans and a red tee-shirt. Her hair is brushed away from her forehead, her eyes look directly at me.

"Oh, yes. She is a lovely lady. Two children of her own. And this is her second time with us. She birthed for us two years ago and is ready to do it again," says Charles. I picture her getting into her station wagon, throwing a toy into the backseat, putting the key into the ignition, and driving off to the nearest IVF clinic to be inseminated with Ed's sperm. All in a day's work. Once I saw a bumper sticker that said: "Happiness is capability." How supremely capable she must feel to dispense such gifts.

Charles tells us more about finding surrogates. He places ads in newspapers in different parts of the country, and he and Connie travel to meet the applicants personally. The next step is a series of intensive interviews. Connie, a clinical psychologist, designed a battery of psychological tests to determine unconscious motivation and screen out women who might have a difficult time after the birth. "We're very thorough with our screening," says Charles. "The most important part of this process is choosing the birth mother. Everything else hinges on that. We reject ninety percent of the applicants. In the last four years not one of the birth mothers in our program has changed her mind. We've arranged eleven births so far."

The combination of having to consider surrogacy as an option, the self-assured manner of our host, and my natural tendency toward paranoia make me a less than courteous client. I interrupt Charles, impatient to proceed. "What are some of the questions you ask in your interviews and where do you place the ads?"

Ed takes my hand. "Why don't we save our questions till after we hear the rest," he says with a "give me a break" look.

Charles drapes his jacket over his chair and loosens his tie. "We advertise mostly in smaller local papers. The questions are designed to determine emotional stability, character, and motivation. Some challenge the woman to think about possible outside pressures. For example, we ask her, 'What would you do if your mother said, I don't want you to give up my grandchild, I'll help you raise her?' If the applicant is married we interview the husband, or any other family member. We want to make sure the birth mother has a strong support system.

"It's important for us to know what makes each woman choose to bear a child for someone else," continues Charles. "Some of them know about the pain of infertility through a friend or a relative. Some have unresolved feelings about having had an abortion or having given up a child for adoption when they were younger. Surrogacy is a way for them to work through their traumas. One young woman was told that a pregnancy could help cure her endometriosis and prevent her own infertility.

"Of course, there are some women who want the money for a new computer or a car. The average fee for our services is twenty-four thousand dollars, out of which ten thousand goes to the surrogate. The money is definitely a

factor, but I strongly feel it should not be the most important one."

Twenty-four thousand dollars? I expected a high fee, but
not this high. I feel a familiar pang of guilt. None of this
would be happening if not for me.

"Do we participate in the interview process?" asks Ed.

"You can, if you choose to. Your relationship with the
surrogate is totally up to you," says Charles. "Some people
prefer no personal contact. On the other end of the spec-
trum is a couple who had the surrogate live with them for
the last month of pregnancy."

I'm still thinking about the money and feel myself getting angry. It's not just the fee. I'm not so open these days
to anyone who tells me how much I need them, how helpless I am on my own. I want to challenge this self-assured
man who knows which woman would change her mind
and keep the baby. Knows what questions to ask and has
them tightly locked away in a drawer full of questionnaires.

I strain for a friendlier tone, but my attitude is not entirely grateful. As I hand him the three hundred dollar
check for the consultation, Charles remarks, "That's for
Erica, my assistant." What he means is, the real money
doesn't come in until we sign a contract.

"No, that's for you," I hear myself saying.

He smiles and gets up from his chair. "Why don't I drive
you to the station."

But we have forty-five minutes before the next train,
and we need the air.

"If it ever does come to this, we'll find our own surrogate," says Ed. I hold on tightly to his arm.

"I can't imagine he would want to work with me. No matter how much we paid him," I say.

It would be an interesting nine months, I muse on the way home. I see myself calling our birth mother every morning to find out what she plans for lunch. Suggest a large organic salad with lots of greens to boost her folic acid? Send a care package with almonds and cashews, some sunflower seeds? A case of organic apple juice? How would I feel about Ed being so intimately connected with another woman? Humiliated? Jealous? It could be a long and winding road, but there would be a baby waiting at the end of it.

I file away the reading material and the copy of the contract we got from Charles. Someday I may reach in the back of the file cabinet and retrieve it. Right now I have no time to waste. The juice bar at Health Nuts is open, and I need a shot of something strong. Like grass.

11

ONE MORE
SPECIALIST

Pay attention to your dreams,
for they are your letters from God.

—Jewish proverb

*I*t's dawn. I'm walking through a deserted Riverside
Park toward the playground. The playground is
empty except for an elderly woman standing near the swings
in a knee-length black dress with a white lace collar and a
round narrow brimmed black hat. She turns to me with a
hint of a smile and I see that she has the deep brown eyes
of my father's sister, only she is much older than my aunt
Adele ever got to be. "Hol van a sapkad? Where is your
hat?" she asks in Hungarian. "Nagy it a szel. It's windy
out here." She motions toward the black rubber seat of the
swing. I can feel the softness of her touch against my back,
and suddenly I understand why she is here. She was sent to
tell me I had passed the test, as did my mother and my
grandmother before me. We had proved that nothing means

more to us than the lives of our children. That we would not trade them for the greatest riches on earth.

"You have to find a prince, a true prince among all the impostors," she says in Hungarian. My feet reach for the ground as I try to get off the swing to face her, but she's gone. I'm in a labyrinth of examining rooms. Men and women in lab coats are rushing through corridors, their faces are expressionless and pale, almost transparent. They belong to a new hybrid species programmed to make as much money as they can. They're looking at my chart. They know that if they point me toward the right trail, I'll get to my destination, but their job is to keep me from getting pregnant. I sneak into their laboratory and pretend to go along with their recommendations, but I'm testing them. I secretly listen to their deliberations, hoping to find the one genuine human who will value life over money. If I can find him, or her, I'll be saved.

I wake up with a sinking feeling of having been betrayed, drenched in sweat, my heart racing. The clock radio says it's three in the morning. The dream hovers over me in the silence of the hour.

A frightening idea comes: I've put my life into the wrong hands and almost lost it. I know it's not true. This is not a life-threatening illness I'm going through. Yet the depth of the betrayal feels like someone has almost succeeded in murdering me. The next feeling is fear. What if I am the traitor? The one who is trespassing? What if I'm

126 acting against some sacred primal law, interrupting a pre-
destined sequence of events? The fear nails me to the bed.
I lie as still as I can, afraid to make the wrong move, as if I
had only this moment to decide whether to keep going or
accept the verdict of the specialists.

But the nightmare is a catalyst for a realization. I'm certain that I can get pregnant again.

After the consultation Ed and I had at the IVF clinic last
year, I accepted the fact that no matter how many doctors I
saw, the answer would remain the same. For eight months,
I have stuck to my self-prescribed treatment, and I'm at
peace with it. But now I'm ready to try just one more specialist.

My friend Lisa still attends Resolve workshops. At the
last meeting she heard of someone who had a high FSH and
was successfully treated by a well-known specialist.

"Do you know how high her FSH was? How old was
she?" I ask, wondering if he is using some new technique.
Lisa doesn't know any of the details, but I've caught the
scent and I'm off and running.

The word is that Dr. D is very thorough and very ex-
pensive. But if he does help me, wouldn't that be worth any
amount?

Maybe I am the one who is being tested. I need to see
him even if it's another dead end. I need to prove to myself
that I'm not like the hybrid species in my dream, and that
his high fee, though much more than I would like to spend,
means nothing to me. I make an appointment for the beginning of August.

It's July 16, Ed's great-aunt's ninety-third birthday. I celebrate it by getting my period. I'm disappointed but, amazingly, I'm able to see it as just another step in the process. Over the last couple of months, I've noticed something remarkable. After six months on my new diet, my menstrual blood turned a bright pink instead of the darkish red it was before. The flow is heavier. I'm bleeding for five days. I remember two of the Chinese healers telling me that the herbs were to lighten the color and increase the flow. My treatment protocol is definitely having an effect! Not quite what I hoped for, but my body is responding.

On August 10, the air-conditioned crosstown bus takes me to my eleven o'clock appointment. Dr. D's spotlessly clean waiting area has the feel of a family living room after dinner. The lighting is subdued. A sofa with a rectangular antique coffee table and a couple of comfortable armchairs. Two elegantly dressed women are seated on the sofa. Their identical hairstyles make the similarity of their features even more striking. But more than that, the older woman's anguished expression, the angle of her head as she turns toward the younger one, give them away as mother and daughter. I discreetly pick up a magazine, but the mother's insistent tone travels across the room: "So ask him. You can ask him anything you want. You're paying him enough."

Internally I find myself defending Dr. D's astronomical fees. He charges as much as he feels he deserves. Perhaps that frees him from selling unnecessary treatments just to hike up his profit. Making the initial fee so high in some way might keep him more honest.

A tall, bearded man about my age gets up from behind a vast desk: "Hi, Bernard D," he says, casually shaking my hand.

He is not terribly happy with my FSH numbers but there has been some fluctuation recently. Maybe they'll keep going down.

"And we should check a couple of more things, just to be sure," he says. On a piece of paper, he carefully charts out several tests not yet included in my fertility workup. One of them is a test for the presence of bacteria that can affect both the quality of the egg as well as the implantation.

"I recently got a call from a woman in Brooklyn," he says, looking pleased, "whom I treated for the very same problem. She was very excited. She said to me, 'Bernie, I didn't think it could happen, but I'm pregnant.' We treated her with antibiotics and it worked." His face is very animated as he tells me this. I have an image of him shouting "Yeah!" then high-fiving the nurses with each positive pregnancy test.

He listens intently to my account of the last two years. The changes in my diet, wheatgrass juice. "I don't know anything about it. What's the juice? It can't hurt."

But I am looking for a little more validation. "My menstrual blood is a lot brighter since I've made these changes, and I have a heavier flow," I say insistently. To press my point further, I add: "It's funny, I might be imagining this, but I feel like I've been having all the symptoms of early pregnancy this month."

He wants to know what exactly I have been feeling.

"Frequent urination. My breasts seem a little more sensitive than usual."

"Let's take a pregnancy test. If we do it right now, we can have the results this afternoon." He gets up and walks me into the examining room.

He draws blood from the vein in my arm into the vial and hands it to the nurse. "Let's get this to the lab before noon."

He turns to me: "You can call the office after four. If it's negative, I want you to do the tests I have outlined for you. If you're pregnant, we'll start you on progesterone as a precautionary measure."

If you're pregnant. He says it so matter-of-factly.

"I don't really think I'm pregnant," I say, wanting to protect both of us from unrealistic expectations.

"Then why did we bother taking a pregnancy test?" he asks with a smirk.

The consultation is over. Although Dr. D didn't come up with any earth-shattering solutions, he didn't seem to feel I was a hopeless case. At least he didn't say so. And he did suggest additional testing. Maybe the tests will reveal something important. I wanted one more specialist and I got him.

Oh, yes, the pregnancy test. I can't possibly take it seriously. Fortunately, I have my afternoon class to bring me back to reality, in case I was even the slightest bit tempted to obsess about it.

I look forward to being with my students. I'm teaching a six-week summer session at the American Language Program at Columbia. My students are young professionals from all over the world: a psychologist from Italy, a German businessman, a Korean journalist, a lawyer from Spain. A lively, generous group.

We're doing one of my favorite lessons, "Close Calls." First, I pretend to almost knock over the bottle of mineral water sitting at the edge of my desk, a trick I've been perfecting for three months. "Now, that was a close call," I say, feigning relief.

The students act out a variation on the theme. Hiroshi, a physicist from Japan, picks up his dictionary and walks straight across the classroom, his head buried in the book. He stops short just as he is about to collide with the blackboard, while the entire class shouts, "Close call!" The students break into small groups to share close call stories.

Each group chooses a story to tell the rest of the class. The result is sometimes moving, sometimes hilarious.

We are all stunned by the account of a young woman lawyer from Madrid. One day she overslept and was driven to school by her father. That afternoon she heard on the news that a terrorist bomb exploded at her usual bus stop at exactly the time she would have ordinarily boarded the bus. After a brief silence, one of the Korean men turns to her and says, "Somebody watching for you up there."

An incredibly handsome, mild-mannered medical student from Germany (on whom all the women in class and at least one teacher have a crush) has a story of nearly wrecking his father's car when he was a teenager, but escaping the accident without a scratch.

Hiroshi is next. "I had to go to the bathroom and I jump out of the boat," he says. "And there was a very big fish. Aaah! I felt deep fear. I don't breathe. But my friend pulled me back in boat. That was lucky experience."

Their anecdotes make Dr. D and babies temporarily recede into the background.

The class is over. It's four o'clock. The results should be in by now. I don't know why my heart should be racing like this. I find the two phones in the faculty lounge. Sherri, another teacher, is on one of the phones. Someone told me earlier today that Sherri is in her first trimester. She is confirming her five-fifteen with Dr. Levi. Must be her obstetrician. A pleading whisper runs through me. This could be me. I could be someone talking to my obstetrician.

"I–N–D–I . . ." says the nurse, looking through the list of lab results. "Oh, yes, Julia, your test came back positive. Well, I guess all you had to do was to see him. Dr. D wants you to take some progesterone. You may not need it. But he wants to be sure. You have to go and pick it up now. I'll give you the address of the drugstore."

What did she say? I am saying something in response. I hear myself laughing. The faculty lounge is suddenly projected onto a screen very far away, and I am alone. The back of my neck vibrates. Placing the phone back on the receiver becomes a task that requires my full concentration. I walk to the bus stop very slowly, gingerly avoiding contact with all animate and inanimate objects, afraid to make any sudden movements, as if I were made of extremely fine crystal. I'm a dancer entrusted with an intricate choreography, I must concentrate and not stumble, take care not to tilt. If I don't follow the dance precisely I will hurt the baby.

I could take a taxi, but the size of the bus seems to afford extra layers of protection. The drugstore is not far from Dr. D's office, and I decide to stop in.

"It looks like we put you in a state of shock," says the nurse with a little laugh. Then she adds, "That backpack looks much too heavy. Why don't you take a taxi and go home? You need to rest."

The trembling inside me subsides. I must call Ed. I make an effort to sound composed, slow down, and not cry. "It's very early," I say, yielding to the madly flashing sign inside my head that reads: DON'T GET TOO EXCITED. PROCEED WITH EXTREME CAUTION.

"You shouldn't go to work," he says. "Just take a taxi and go home. I'll be home early. Take deep breaths, okay?"

I can feel his fragility over the phone. Deliberate slowing down. The fear of making the wrong move. The need to keep his excitement under control, as if both of us now had to be very careful to do the right thing and at the same time not let ourselves feel too deeply how much we want this to be real.

I call the director of the evening program at La Guardia to let him know I can't make tonight's class.

Dr. D wants me to go for a blood test every other day to make sure all the hormone levels are rising as expected. Two weeks later I am scheduled for a first sonogram. I'm too nervous to look at the screen, but Dr. E, the radiologist, confirms it: "There is an early intrauterine gestational sac." She schedules me for a follow-up in two weeks.

Sonogram No. 2: "A slow fetal heartbeat is noted." But the sonogram also reveals a small separation between the placenta and the uterus. Dr. D wants me to take one baby aspirin each day. It's meant to thin my blood and keep my blood flow more even.

On Friday night, a few days after the second sonogram, I start bleeding. I must have miscarried. My body and my face feel swollen as I try to hold in all the feeling. I can't afford to fall apart. I call Dr. D's office. "There is nothing we can do right now," says the nurse. "The lab is closed. Just stay in bed. We'll take a test on Monday." Ed rushes home to be with Ellena.

I have a healing meditations tape I bought at Kripalu, a yoga center we visited in the spring. I lie on my red yoga blanket, taking slow, deep breaths, listening to the gentle voice of Carolyn Lunden, a teacher at the center. The blurb on the cover says she created the tape after her personal experience with cancer.

Monday's blood test says I'm still pregnant. But we are far from the safe zone. The nurse warns me to be cautious: "You must not lift any heavy objects, and you must stay horizontal as much as possible."

My friend Amy and her son Gabriel come over to entertain Ellena. Karen and Sylvia take her to the playground. Ed takes days off from work. I keep listening to Carolyn Lunden's reassuring voice. Every other day, I call the nurse, hoping she will confirm that the hormone levels are normal. And they are. During my next visit to the radiologist, I'm told the chorion-amnion separation is no longer a problem.

I'm in my twelfth week of pregnancy. It's time for the last sonogram. If all is well, I will be leaving Dr. D for an obstetrician. It's the first time I dare look at the monitor. Dr. E points to a dark, pulsating spot on the screen. "That's the heartbeat. It's nice and strong. Congratulations," she says, smiling. Her assistant pats me on the shoulder: "Good luck to you."

There is a phone booth right outside her office. Ed is waiting to hear from me. "Everything is fine," I say. We're both crying. And laughing.

A baby, a person, another member of our family. I'm floating along Eighty-sixth Street, my head buzzing. A ray of color streams out from a store window in congratulatory greeting. I beam at each passerby, silently thanking all of them for letting me have this baby. As if their being here at this very moment is part of a grand scheme that is making it possible. I want to walk up to them and say: "Guess what? It happened. It really happened. I'm going to have a baby."

The funny thing is that everyone seems to be smiling at me. They must think I'm in love. And I am, in love with the emerging life inside me. The way it made its way from the darkness of FSH numbers and over-forty statistics. The way it sailed right past the dignified Park Avenue offices and clinics with a list of prerequisites, none of which included taking better care of one's body and soul.

What would they say to me now, the long line of re-spected, even famous, experts in the field? They pro-nounced me doomed by my FSH. They suggested IVF, egg donors, Pergonal. "I'm sorry," they intoned. "There is nothing you can do." It's the finality of their diagnosis, the certainty of their voices, the grave faces and the folded hands that made me walk out of their offices numb and stripped of hope. "There must be someone out there that conceived with these numbers, just one person?" I pleaded.

"Sorry," they replied emphatically. "No one."

The month Ed and I, with the help of a benevolent uni-verse, ignited the spark of Adira's life, my FSH was 30.4. "Let's just go to sleep," I said on production night. "It's no use this month." But Ed is a believer.

"So this is a miracle baby," says Dr. Moss, my obstetri-cian, after going over my records. Under his watchful eye, I have six more months of an uneventful pregnancy.

My daughter, Adira Indich Baum, is born a week after my due date, on April 29, 1994.

12

LESSONS FROM ADI

Kicsi a bors, de eros.
Small is the peppercorn, but strong.

— a Hungarian proverb

Adi is now two and a half years old. She makes her own morning cocktail. Her favorite part is placing the carrot into the juicer, then using her entire body weight to press it through the chute.

All of us are still on a modified vegetarian diet. I passed on the two red yoga blankets to Ellena and Adi and got two blue ones for me and Ed. At the moment, our group practice sessions are pretty tightly controlled by Ellena, but Adi will soon be contributing her own repertoire of original poses.

I make time to do my yoga practice and meditation each day, even if just for half an hour. Overall, I continue with all the adjustments in my diet and lifestyle which helped me get pregnant.

Once in a while, I get nostalgic for a piece of chocolate

cake with buttercream icing or a large plate of french fries
with ketchup, and sometimes I give in to the temptation.
But whenever I think about the variety of junk food I used
to assault my body with on a daily basis, I'm thankful for
the wake-up call. I'm thankful not just for the astounding
gift of Adi's presence, but also for the gifts she brought with
her.

Though I was unaware of it at the time, this journey was
more about learning to believe in myself than about getting
pregnant. It was the first time in my life I dared to follow
through on all the healthy impulses that urged me to keep
going.

In 1984, visiting Czechoslovakia for the first time after
fifteen years in America, I called John S, one of my old
classmates from the University of Performing Arts. He was
now an internationally known theater and television director. "Oh, Julia!" he exclaimed, "Julia the promising actress." "Promising." The word made me wince with shame.
Promising and never realized. Adi, before I ever saw her
face, showed me I could be someone who doesn't turn
back. She rallied the rebel forces inside me. She helped me
understand that although I may not always achieve the result I aim for, I must still act on what I believe in.

She taught me to recognize the destroyers in my life, the
people who can't resist poking a finger into my tower of
blocks and watch them scatter all over the floor. The "real-
ists" who stand by with a list of a hundred rational reasons
not to disrupt the pattern of acceptable solutions.

I sometimes dream of my half brother, Robika. In one

dream, I am sitting on a tricycle. He pushes me up a steep hill, his hands on my back. I realize now that my yearning for another child was also a yearning for Robika and all the other relatives that crowded the stories of my childhood, leaving an empty space. I see Adi and Ellena as a continuation of their interrupted lives.

My children have helped me to finally acknowledge my rage over the injustices visited on my family. After all these years, my rage doesn't seem to subside. After forty years it still informs my decisions and my daily reality. Now I let it be my fuel instead of turning it against myself.

With my daughter leading the way I have learned the perils of title worship. Before she came along, I usually needed someone with the proper credentials to validate my experience. In my willingness to abdicate all decision-making to my physicians, I was not unlike a colleague of mine who, after six years of unexplained infertility, continues to drink her daily cups of coffee, her glasses of wine, and smoke her allowance of cigarettes, all because the man with the "M.D." behind his name says it's okay.

Before Adira came along, it never occurred to me to challenge my doctors' advice. When they said, "There is nothing you can do," I assumed that was the truth. A few days before my due date, my cervix was not softening, and I was afraid I would have to have a second cesarean section. I asked one of the physicians who examined me if there was anything I could do to help things along. "Nothing," he said. "If there is no change in the next week, we can give you an injection of prostaglandin."

After a little investigation among my circle of subversive informers, I found that semen contained the same chemical as the drug. I decided I'd much rather have it in its natural form, and I figured out just where I could get it. Ed had no objection to this form of intervention. I also started doing specific imaging exercises to make my cervix more receptive. The result: the transformation of my cervix from stubborn to willing.

I was lucky that my doctors knew of no current technology that could fix me, or I would have kept going for more and more exotic treatments. Just about every speaker at every presentation I went to emphasized that the age of the egg determines the ability to conceive and sustain a pregnancy. "Once your ovaries show signs of decline," they said, "it's time for drugs."

Not one of the mainstream specialists suggested that nourishing the body, getting rid of toxins in my food, taking advantage of the physiological benefits of specific exercises, or diving in for a bit of psychological exploration might reverse the diagnosis.

As a child, I heard a Hungarian folktale. There was once a very sad and frail princess. The merest gust of cool air made her cough and take to bed with fever. The king and queen promised half the kingdom to anyone who would save their daughter, Anna. Healers from far away mixed their potions and cast their spells. The princess remained sickly and inconsolable.

Then one day, just when it looked like the poor girl was going to wither away, a peasant from the nearby village showed up at the castle. "My name is Barna Janos," he said to the king, "and I came to cure the princess." He brought a wagon full of vegetables and fruits from his farm. He prescribed lots of sunshine and fresh air. He invited some children from the village to teach her their games. Within a month the princess was ready to live happily ever after. "You're only a simple peasant. How did you know you could heal our daughter?" asked the queen. "I didn't," said Janos. "But I would have been a fool not to try."

For many of us, taking action may not be so simple. Results may not show up as quickly as for princess Anna. Yet, the alternative is waiting for the next instructions from our doctors, the way we wait by the phone for the call that never comes.

The most difficult part for me was finding the tiny crack of possibility in the wall of "expert certainty." Then I discovered more and more cracks, until the wall turned into a rickety fence with a hole large enough to squeeze through. Helpers were waiting on the other side. They gave no guarantees, but they showed me the power of doing my share of the work.

We're at the playground. Ellena can hardly contain her pride in her sister, the little person marching beside her: "Come, Adi, come. You wanna go on the slide? Yeah?" I extend a protective arm to catch the little one as she leans over the side. "No, I'm watching her," says the big sister. And she is. She also squeezes her, and hugs and picks her up

and sometimes squeezes a little too hard and sometimes   *141*
screams in frustration because "Adi messed up my things."

Seeing them together, I'm reminded of a colleague's remark as she watched me devour a piece of *dhuri* fruit, an al-
leged fertility booster. "Ugh, it's just not worth it," she said,
feigning nausea. Oh, yes it is. It's worth every single bite.

13

LETTERS FROM THE FRONT

When Adi was six months old and our lives had settled in, I asked my friend Amy, a seasoned journalist, to help me tell our story. "Just put down what you remember, and we'll take it from there," said Amy. After she read the first draft, she cheered me on to finish the project myself, adding her sharp-eyed editing.

The article was turned down by four publications ("Sorry, we're not doing infertility right now"), but friends suggested turning it into a book. I wrote four chapters.

Literary agents and editors responded that, although the writing was engaging, I lacked the proper credentials. The market was already flooded with books by specialists, they said, and since what I underwent was secondary infertility, many women would not read the story since my pain was not as deep as theirs. "And it's not like you're somebody famous," said one editor before he hung up.

One day, reading yet another rejection letter, it struck me that this was Adi's story all over again. Once again, someone was predicting that my efforts would be futile. This time, I had a blueprint to follow. If I didn't finish this book, I would have learned nothing from my "miraculous conception."

I began going to Resolve meetings to remind myself why I was writing and to make the connections I was afraid to make four years earlier. I usually just sat and listened, or exchanged stories with the person sitting next to me.

The topic of one of the support groups was secondary infertility. It was the first time I had the courage to speak up. I told the dozen or so women and men around the large conference table that I was compelled to come to meetings even though I was no longer trying to get pregnant, and I told them about my book. No one asked me to leave. The warm welcome of the facilitator made me realize I had more healing to do.

Janet and Anne, two women I met at the meeting, read the sample chapters and urged me to continue. I felt I must write as fast as I could. At three in the morning I scribbled into the notebook near my pillow, or I stopped in the middle of the street to jot down a line before it slipped away.

As the project progressed, I discovered seminars on Chinese medicine, herbal walks, and workshops on natural healing methods. In these forays, I found another group of fierce enthusiasts who had success stories with a holistic approach to various ailments, including reproductive problems.

Listening to them, I remembered the accountant of hope that sat on my shoulders six years ago keeping close count of every success and failure. The failures could make me slide back into depression, the successes set me zooming ahead like "the little engine who could."

So here are the stories of five of the women I met: Carol, Sallie, Laura, Marie, and Ellen. Meeting them was yet another of Adi's gifts.

Carol, New York, New York ▪ *Livia, 6 lb. 8 oz.*

I think the most significant thing about my history is that I waited for a long time to have a child because of my professional dance career.

I was thirty-nine when Brad and I started having unprotected sex. After two years, I still wasn't pregnant. One of my clients went through two IVF pregnancies, and I was her personal trainer through both of them. She urged me to see her doctor and to get some preliminary tests.

I liked Dr. M a lot. He was good to talk to. He really listened to what I had to say and was not on a power kick. First he checked my hormone levels. He reassured me that I was not going into menopause. He did a hysterosalpingogram, and my tubes were clear. The postcoital test was next. What he found was that there were no sperm in the uterus, not even dead sperm. Dr. M explained that sometimes they find a lot of dead sperm which indicates that there is a negative climate present. But no sperm at all? He was very surprised. My husband's sperm count was good, there was good motility. Yet the sperm were not making it past the cervical mucus. He didn't really know why this was happening, and at that point, he said I couldn't get pregnant without intervention.

The first procedure we did was intrauterine insemination. At a specified time, they took a sonogram to see if the follicles were mature, and then after I released the egg they put the concentrated sperm right in the uterus. I thought, "This is going to do it."

It didn't work. We tried it once more, and again it didn't work. Then Dr. M said, "Let's try a little Clomid." This time there were three mature follicles, and I really had my hopes up. We tried Clomid with intrauterine insemination for a couple of more cycles. When that didn't work, Dr. M started talking about IVF.

Maybe I would have done it, because I was really hooked in. He was connected with a fertility clinic, and in the waiting room there was a whole thick scrapbook of pictures of babies, mostly twins, with inscriptions, "Thank you, Dr. M." I was tempted. But I had accumulated a large bill because he allowed me to just pay as much as I could. The inseminations were five hundred dollars a shot, and I still owed him a couple of thousand dollars.

My husband, who was never very keen on the whole thing, finally put his foot down. He wanted a child, but he felt if it was going to happen, it was going to happen. He didn't want to go any further with medical intervention.

At first I panicked. I thought, Oh, no, maybe this means

I'm never going to have any children. Then I started talking to my friends about it and wondering what else could I do. A colleague of mine was studying Chinese medicine and taking Tai Chi with a man in Riverside Park. He told her about a Chinese doctor who had just come over from China.

It was very hard to communicate with Clopin at first. She was in the back room of a pharmacy in Chinatown. The owner was a grim-looking man. There were pig's feet and all sorts of strange things around. She took my pulse, looked at my tongue, and asked me a lot of questions about my periods and my bowel movements. She said I had a weak liver. She had me go back to taking my temperature and charting my ovulation, and she gave me herbs that were meant to tone various systems. Some of them were for thinning of the mucus, which started making a lot of sense to me. I used to wear contact lenses and at some point couldn't wear them anymore. I had had all kinds of eye exams and was told that there was too much mucus in my tears. So I just had this feeling that maybe the same situation existed in my vagina. The sperm couldn't make it through the thick mucus even though the motility test was okay.

They were quite vile, the herbs Clopin gave me. They smelled up the house, but I kept mixing and drinking them according to her instructions. Around the strategic time she did intensive acupuncture. I would be there for an hour and a half with needles in me. By this time, I was forty-one. Clopin was in her twenties, and she later admitted that she thought I was too old. So I think she was doing all she could. I really did feel a change from the herbs. I felt stronger and more stimulated.

At the time, I was also involved with a spiritual group, led by a woman named Julie Kane. She has a background in nursing. She did a lot of counseling through Columbia University, and then she broke away from that. The work I did with her individually was similar to psychotherapy. But she would also make me tea and she did some reflexology. She came to my house.

When I first started working with her, I lived in this little place and I was very driven. As a choreographer, I was producing my concerts, and I was always on the run. My home was just a place to come sleep and sublet if I was going away. Julie wanted me to embellish my home, helped me make it more comfortable. She helped me discover what my belief systems were and how they were working against me.

She invited me to join a spiritual support group. My work with them was very helpful when I was trying to get pregnant. Everyone in the group—there were eight of us—was very supportive. At some point, we started doing affirmations for each other every day. We were all working on something. People had career goals or health issues, and each of us wrote out an affirmation for ourselves and for the other people in the group. We all did them every night at the same time. I still remember mine: "Under God's grace and perfect ways, Mother Father God, I have received this sperm into my body to create a union with an

148 egg within me. The beautiful, perfect child is now being brought into being through radiant light and love. Brad and I welcome this child through unconditional love, great mind, and joy. Thank you, Universe." I started doing this affirmation six months before I met Clopin.

There was this positive mental energy going out every day for me. There was a lot of power in that.

Two months after I started working with Clopin, I was going to be on a tour in upstate New York. So I said, forget about this month because I was going to be gone exactly around the time when we should've been trying. I drank the teas the first week of the cycle and then she gave me herbs in a pill form. She even gave me some herbs for Brad. I went on the gig, and Brad came up to see the performance. We spent a few days in our country house after the tour. The next month my period was late, but that has happened a few other times. When we did the inseminations my period was once eight days late. So I thought it was the same thing again. I also thought it couldn't be this month because we weren't together during the fertile time.

A few days later we went to visit Brad's parents, and our car broke down. We got a ride home with his mother. I remember we were having breakfast someplace, and I felt a little queasy. I thought, this is strange. By this time, I was ten days late. When we got home, I got a pregnancy test from the drugstore, and it was positive! I was completely shocked. After all I had been doing, all that planning and then just to have this bizarre timing. I had a very good pregnancy, very good birth. No intervention at all.

Doing the herbs Clopin gave me addressed some systems in my body that needed fortifying or toning, though I was quite skeptical when I first went to see her. I noticed some definite changes in my energy level. The herbs also helped with my allergies. I certainly did not believe in Chinese medicine as much as I believed in the intrauterine inseminations. My father was a general practitioner back in the old days. He thought even chiropractors were quacks, and I did have that seed of distrust in me.

On the other hand, having led a bohemian lifestyle, I had been exposed to alternative ways of thinking. I wasn't a ballerina in the studio smoking cigarettes; I was a modern dancer who did groovy things. I went to graduate school in California in the '70s, and we were involved in all sorts of bodywork techniques, like rolfing, Feldenkreis, and Alexander. I studied the Bartinia fundamentals, which are based on integrating mind and body. So, luckily, even though a part of me was skeptical, I was open to explore other options.

Sallie, Woodstock, New York ▪ *Noah, 8 lb. 13 oz.*

I was thirty-five when I met my husband, Steve. We were neighbors. We lived in this funky old walk-up, and one day, he helped me carry my packages in. A friend of mine was staying with me for a few days, and after he left she said, "There's a great guy for you."

I said to her, "Please, I hardly know his name." Later,

when I did find out a little about him, I thought, oh, right, this is really what I need! He is seven years younger than me. No thank you! He is an actor. No thank you. But my friend was right. His age was not a consideration, once I got to know him. I thought it would've been more of an issue for him, but it wasn't. Except that he was a little worried about the idea of kids, because I was thirty-five, and he felt he was not ready for children. He came to New York to make it as an actor, and the last thing he wanted to do was to strap himself down.

Three years later, after we got married, and I started edging toward forty, getting pregnant became more of a pressure. I was nervous about it because so many people around me were having problems. I was with a group of midwives (this was long before I even thought of getting pregnant) for my well-care and they also told me I should start as soon as possible.

We actually got pregnant the first time we tried. I was thirty-nine. We went to the midwives and the test was positive. We had a big two-hour visit with them. It was very exciting. They put us in touch with a group of women gynecologists that they used for amnios.

Dr. H was very nice. She spent a lot of time talking to us about risk factors. And then she said, "Let's do an ultrasound and see how far along you are." We did. It was clearly a blighted ovum that I hadn't released yet.

That was very traumatic. We had already told family and some friends. But Dr. H was a remarkably healing doctor. She said, "Don't worry. It's a good sign that you got pregnant so fast." As we were waiting to go in for the D&C (the scraping) she was holding my hand, and we talked about books and music. She helped us turn a traumatic situation into a healing event. I felt very turned around by it.

We started trying again soon after, and we were having problems. I cried every time I got my period. I started charting my ovulation. It seemed I was taking my temperature every five minutes. This went on for over a year. Steve was getting a little impatient, and one day, after I got my period, he said we should go and talk to Dr. H and have some tests. We did a semen analysis for him. But somehow, every time I scheduled a test for me, something came up and I ended up canceling the appointment.

I resisted going the medical route. I had friends that did a lot of intervention, and I saw some of them getting very angry and bitter about the whole process. I wanted to, if at all possible, stay out of that cycle.

Then one day, my friend Mark, a pediatrician, said to me, "I've heard of Diane D, a craniosacral therapist who has been very successful with infertility problems." He explained that the treatment was based on the idea that the body functions as a closed hydraulic structure and blockages can create organ or immune system dysfunction. The therapist uses a gentle hands-on approach to remove those blocks. Mark knew one of Diane's patients personally. She got pregnant after two years of trying. He handed me Diane's card. I have a very clear memory of Mark telling me this. Something in me went, This is it.

When I first went to Diane, she asked a lot of questions

about my history. Not medical history but emotional history, difficulties in my past, any unresolved issues that I felt might be blocking me emotionally. That's very much part of the work.

During the session, Diane would touch various points on my head. Sometimes she was even inside my mouth, gently pressing on the roof of my mouth. Or she would touch points near my ovaries. Most of the time I was very quiet. I was there for an hour and a half and often I said very little.

Then one day, I said something, as she touched a point near my temples, and I started to cry. I think my work with Diane helped release a great deal of emotional and physical stress. Stuff that had been there for a long time and got stirred up by the pressures of the previous year.

I saw her once a week, and my body started changing after just a few sessions. My periods changed. The color of blood was strikingly different. Much more vivid. I also started having unbelievable dreams about babies. In one dream there was an image of a bull's-eye and then a baby flowing out of it.

One weekend, about two months after I had started my work with Diane, we spent a week at our summer home in Woodstock. I got my period and I was really sad. I asked my friend Susan to take a walk with me around Cooper Lake. The weather had been strange. One day it was really cold and the next day it got warm. The lake was frozen, but it was starting to melt. It was dusk and there was all this steam coming off the lake. We were walking along a little path. On one side of us was a marsh.

Suddenly I looked over and saw a beaver swimming across the lake with a stick in his mouth. As we were watching him, three swans swam into our field of vision. I looked at Susan and I said, "This is my sign." I sat down and wrote it in my journal.

Next month my period was late. I didn't say anything to Steve. He didn't keep such close track of my cycle, he usually just knew by my crying that I got my period. We were up at Woodstock again, and he went out for a run. While he was out, I did one of those home pregnancy tests. When Steve got back, I had it wrapped in a foil with a ribbon on it. I said to him, "I bought this for you, it's just a silly little thing." He was standing there, sweating, and he opened it and there it was.

I had a great pregnancy and an amazing birth.

I remember when I first started seeing Diane, she said to me, "Put away the thermometer, put away the calendar, and just be together." And that was so freeing. That really helped. Not keeping track. It used to make me so uptight.

I work with children and families who have to face tough diagnoses, and I know that it makes all the difference in the world how you approach your treatment and how you approach your body. Whether what you hear from people is sensitivity and caring and belief, or papers and numbers and statistics.

Going through infertility can be such a devastating experience. You are so vulnerable to begin with. You are so much on that precipice of judging yourself completely by what is happening to you. Wanting a baby desperately, as if somehow this is the thing that's going to make you whole. And hating it at the same time. You keep denying that you need it to be whole. You say to yourself, Oh, I don't really need this, it won't really matter if I never have a kid. But I'll spend twenty thousand dollars more to try. That's what a lot of people I know are going through. They are caught up in it. I think you have to be forgiving of yourself, to stop feeling like you failed when things don't work out the way you wish they had.

My work with Diane helped with that, too. I had a lot of very supportive people around me. My friend Susan in Woodstock knew of many women who were having babies later in life. She was never one to listen to statistics. Steve was always very optimistic.

Whom you surround yourself with is very important. I really didn't want to hear anything other than what was going to help me believe in myself. I have strong beliefs about the power of the words we use. If you say to yourself, I can't do it, I can't do it, I can't do it, all day long, it becomes self-fulfilling.

Laura, Nyack, New York ▪ *Susan, 5 lb. 10 oz.*

Jeff and I had been living together for two years when I decided that I wanted to have a baby. We started trying as soon as we got married. Every month I kept look-ing for signs of morning sickness. After breakfast, I would say to Jeff, "Oh, I feel a little nauseous today," and then my period would come, and I would be in tears. It was excru-ciating. Six months later, I went to see my gynecologist just to check if there was anything I should be doing. She did a routine gynecological exam and said that everything was fine.

"You're only thirty-four, and you haven't been trying that long. Relax," she said.

After six more months of trying, I made an appointment to see a specialist at NYU. There was a two-month wait to see him.

Earlier that year, I had had an experience which got me interested in the medicinal use of herbs. For our honey-moon, Jeff and I had gone camping in the Barrens, and a week after we came home I got an intensely itchy rash all over my legs. My foot swelled up to twice its normal size, and I couldn't walk on it. I went to the doctor and she said, "You're having an allergic reaction to something." She also said that my foot was infected and gave me some antibiotics and some cortisone cream for the rash. Both of these sounded scary to me. I had a lot of allergies, and I was afraid the antibiotics would mess up my system. The cream didn't feel like a good thing either.

I went to Angelica herb store and I looked through a number of books. In *Back to Eden,* which is a classic herbal text by Jethro Kloss, he tells a story of somebody with an infected foot.

He said one should soak the foot alternately in hot and cold water, then soak it in kerosene. I didn't have any kerosene, so for the last soak I put some echinacea tincture into the water. I knew that echinacea is good for infections of any kind. If this doesn't work in a week, I said to myself, I'll take the antibiotics. The next morning more than half of the swelling was gone. I could walk. It made such an impression on me that I thought, One of these days I'll have to learn more about this.

It seemed that now was the time to find out what herbs could do for me. I got Susun Weed's book called *Wise Woman Herbal for the Childbearing Year*. It's mainly about herbs for pregnancy with a short section on fertility. I had already been drinking herbal teas, but I got a lot more serious about it.

Her method of preparation is to fill a jar one-third to one-half full with the herbs, then pour boiling water in it and let it steep for four hours. It comes out pretty strong. A cup of that a day is a substantial amount.

Susun's favorite herb for establishing fertility is red clover. It's meant to alkalize the system, make it more hospitable to sperm. It also has estrogenic precursors that the body can use to build estrogen. I drank red clover once or twice a week.

I was more drawn to nettles and raspberry leaf. Nettles are specifically a blood-builder, high in iron and calcium. The interesting thing about nettles is that they support the liver. In Chinese medicine, the liver stores the blood, and it needs to work well to make the blood healthy.

The raspberry leaf tea is a uterine tonic. It strengthens the uterus and the whole reproductive system.

I alternated those three infusions and drank a cup of something every day. Drinking the teas felt very nourishing, like eating vegetables that were just picked out of a garden. As I was drinking, I thought, Wow, this is really good for me.

My diet was already fairly good, but as I was learning more about plants, I ate more edible weeds, like dandelion greens, lamb's quarters, and chickweed. I went to Prospect Park and picked them myself, which made me feel an emotional connection with them. I didn't just go down the street and pay money for them. I interacted with them. It has given me a whole different dimension of experiencing nature. I discovered that nature was not just something you could go and look at. I experienced myself as a part of the food chain. I drank nettles. Then the mosquitoes drank my blood; the birds ate the mosquitoes and fertilized the plants. Being connected to what goes on in nature became part of the healing process for me.

I got so involved in studying herbs that I decided to cancel my appointment with the specialist, partly because I found out that it was going to cost hundreds of dollars and partly because of my horror of doctors. I kept drinking my teas.

A friend I met in one of my herb classes was taking a course in acupressure. It's similar to acupuncture, but instead of needles, you use your fingers. To practice, we worked on each other for hours.

I had also been meditating at least an hour a day, trying to get more in touch with the spiritual part of me. One month, I was really convinced I was pregnant. My breasts were more tender, I was nauseous, and I had to urinate more frequently. Then I got my period, and that was devastating because I'd been so sure about it. I thought, How could this happen? Not only wasn't I pregnant, I was wrong. I felt that I couldn't trust my intuition.

I recovered and kept reading. One of the books on getting pregnant talked about how it often happens that an egg can be fertilized but it won't implant in the uterus, particularly if the uterine lining isn't thick enough. I realized I was probably pregnant when I thought I was—my hormones were changing—but I couldn't hold on to the egg.

I went back to Susun Weed's book and learned about false unicorn root, which has been used for centuries for fertility. Susun calls it a uterine tonic, with an alkalizing influence on the ovaries, kidneys, and bladder. When I asked an herbalist friend about it, he said that estrogenic compounds circulate through the body and the body has receptor sites, particularly on the ovaries, where estrogen is needed for ovulation. The receptors have to match the structure of the particular estrogen that they're going to pick up. False unicorn enables the receptors to work, which facilitates the ovaries' taking in the estrogen. This sounded very useful to me.

I knew that when you are using herbs specifically for hormonal balance, you should start around the time you ovulate and take them until you menstruate, but I needed to do something right away. I bought false unicorn root in a tincture form and started taking it two days after I got my period. I took it for the whole month.

I got pregnant the following month. Of course, I had been drinking the teas for two years, and I felt a gradual change in my energy level, but I do feel that the false unicorn root contributed in readying my body.

In retrospect, I feel lucky that my gynecologist didn't pressure me into anything. I was brought up to have a tremendous respect for doctors, and it induces a passive attitude in me. It's very difficult for me to question them. Had she recommended some sophisticated treatment, I'm not sure what I would have done. I was getting quite desperate.

It was very gratifying to navigate through the experience on my own. It has made me feel like a stronger person.

Marie, Portland, Oregon ■ *Lucy, 7 lb. 3 oz.*

I got married in Florida when I was twenty-seven. I'm a biologist, my husband is an economist. We traveled all over the place. I was happy with my career and my marriage, and I didn't want to have kids at all.

At some point, I got a new female boss, who drove me crazy. All I had to do was walk by her office and I'd get a knot in my stomach. It was the strangest thing—she pushed all my buttons. That's when I started to feel a need to understand myself better.

One day I tuned in to John Bradshaw on public television. I read his book and lots of other self-help books. I started to figure out that maybe the idea of not wanting to have kids had to do with things in my past.

My own childhood was miserable. I didn't want to bring anybody else into the world that I would treat the way I was treated. My parents were children and I'd spent my whole life trying to meet their needs and never succeeded because they were just insatiable. The idea of introducing somebody else into my life that depended on me was suffocating.

My husband never pressured me to have kids. I found out later that he told other people that he would like to have children, but he never pushed me. He wanted me to be the one who initiated it.

Something inside me said that I was probably going to miss out on this wonderful experience. But I'm a scientist by nature, I'm into data, facts. Things had to make sense to me.

Through my reading and through working with a therapist, it became clear that my reasons for not wanting to have children were based on things that didn't exist anymore.

I started trying to get pregnant when I was thirty-six. I was trying and trying, and every month I would go through that horrible emotional exhaustion. After six months my doctor suggested I start charting my ovulation. I did that. I moved on to an ovulation kit and it still didn't work.

Finally, I got pregnant and I was elated. I was surprised

that I didn't feel any nausea or fatigue, but my doctor said that some women just had an easier time than others.

We went on vacation and I woke up in the middle of the night with cramps. My doctor told me to fly home, and they did an ultrasound. There was no heartbeat, but they said it might just be too early, and they told me to stay in bed for a week. It was very hard. At the end of the week the ultrasound showed no pregnancy.

They detected a fibroid on the outside of my uterus, but they said it had nothing to do with the miscarriage.

It was a shock to learn that just because you're pregnant, it doesn't mean you're going to have a baby. It was as if someone had played a bad joke on me.

I waited about two months, and I got pregnant again really quickly. I miscarried two days later.

My doctor suggested doing an endometrial biopsy.

When the tests came back, Dr. S said that my progesterone levels were low, and I should take progesterone suppositories. I said to myself these people are the experts; I know nothing about this.

I tried the suppositories for a couple of months, and then I stopped. I just didn't feel good about it. It was extremely frustrating.

At that point, I talked to my cousin, who said she had heard about a homeopath in New York. My cousin was the one who got me into therapy, and she has always turned me on to good things.

The first time I called Karen, the homeopath, I asked her to explain to me what she did. She told me that homeopathy had been around for two hundred years, and was based on the principle of treating like with like. "It's a little like a vaccination," she said. She also talked about changing the body's energy field and vital force. It was all really foreign to me. Skeptic that I was, I just wasn't at all sure.

Karen asked me to write her a letter about myself, about any emotional and physical traumas, anything that I felt had shaped me. And I sent her a picture of myself. Then we had a two-hour phone consultation, which was very emotional. It was such a relief to talk to her. I just wanted someone to care about my problem, and to give me hope.

Homeopathic medicine uses highly diluted remedies made from natural substances. They're prescribed on the basis of a myriad of characteristics: your likes and dislikes, your attitude toward things, and a wide range of stimuli.

Karen gave me a remedy called pulsatilla. Pulsatilla is a wild flower that bends with the wind. It was appropriate, she said, for people who were sensitive, and had a hard time making decisions. I had to put it in water and then take a sip a couple of times a day. Six weeks later, I had another session with Karen. I felt much less fragile. She said that I was on the right track, and she wanted me to continue with the same remedy. I conceived six weeks later.

I was afraid to get too excited at first, but then I realized that this was the right pregnancy.

My reading had opened me up intellectually but it was all in my head. The remedy and my work with Karen helped my body to absorb the information as well.

As the pregnancy progressed I continued to talk to her,

and she changed remedies to help me with nausea and anxiety.

At some point during the second trimester, I started feeling claustrophobic. As a child I had had to rely on myself for everything. And it's still really hard for me to give up control. Karen tried very hard to help me with the claustrophobia, and then she hit on argentum. I had to take one pellet twice a day. It worked like magic.

I was also concerned about the fibroid on the outside of my uterus, and I found a book which discussed how emotional issues manifest in the body. It said that people get fibroids when they reject their feminine side, which is what I had been doing for a long time. Not wanting to be associated with my mother in any way, I had cut off my femininity.

I went on a quest to open up my feminine side, and to get into the pregnancy on a spiritual level.

When I first saw my little girl, I felt such a flood of joy. She is two and a half now, and I have a six-months-old baby boy.

Ellen, New York, New York ▪ *Michael, 6 lbs. 5 oz.*

I was thirty-six when I got married, and although I realized that time was of the essence, there was just too much going on for us to start getting pregnant right away. We needed to move, and my husband was in the midst of a career change. Coming from a large family, I knew that

164   children were a great deal of work. I wanted to be sure that I had a partner in parenting.

When we finally decided to start trying, I thought I would get pregnant right away. In my late teens and early twenties, I had gotten pregnant twice, using birth control. In those days my fertility made me nervous. I was very surprised when, after three months, I was not pregnant. I talked to my gynecologist, and she suggested a series of tests. My husband, Steve, had a sperm count taken. We were told that all the tests were fine. There was nothing wrong with either one of us.

I had a college friend who was trying to get pregnant as well. Her cousin, a fertility specialist, was pressuring her to go the high-tech route, and she started pushing me in the same direction.

"I think I'm going to wait," I said to her. I was more interested in finding out why it wasn't working than getting too anxious about starting with procedures.

After four months of working with my gynecologist, I got a specialist. He was one of the doctors listed in my insurance packet, an older man with an office on Park Avenue. He had me chart my ovulation. "You just need to relax," he said. "This is a very chancy thing. You never know when it is going to work." Six months later, I was still not pregnant, and now I started to wonder what was going on. I also noticed that every time I went to see my Park Avenue specialist, the waiting room was filled with older women. He claimed he was a reproductive endocrinologist, but I think he was really an oncologist.

I decided it was time to change doctors, and I made an appointment with Dr. S, a specialist connected with a major IVF clinic. Things looked a lot better there. The first thing Dr. S said after looking through my chart was "We're going to get you pregnant. I don't know what it's going to take, but we'll do it." For a while I was on an upswing.

Up until then, all the attention was on me and my age. Forty, forty. They kept flashing the word in front of me like a big neon sign. But Dr. S scheduled some additional tests for my husband.

In the meantime, they started me out on Clomid and had us do artificial insemination. They said, "Let's go full steam ahead, let's do everything." And at that point I said to myself, It's been a little while, why not do everything? After about a month and a half of tests, they figured out that the penetrating ability of my husband's sperm was the problem. Dr. S told us at that point that we would never get pregnant without IVF.

"It looks like this is much more serious than we thought," Steve said. "We might as well educate ourselves about what's available for us."

Three other couples were at the introductory IVF seminar. The director of the clinic explained the whole procedure. Everyone else was so enthusiastic. One couple from South America was ready to pay cash right there. According to the clinic's success rates, one out of four couples went home with a baby. I looked around the room and thought, Okay, who is it going to be? I became quite anxious after hearing how involved a procedure IVF was. I'm frightened of needles.

Steve and I were very discouraged after that seminar. I started to camouflage my infertility. Our friends knew we were going through treatment, and when they asked how things were going, I would say, "I'm starting to wonder if I would be a good mother." There was also a group of women I had been meeting with every couple of weeks. Two of the women became pregnant. That was difficult for me. One night, there was a shower for one of the women, and I couldn't go. I was all dressed to go and, at the last minute, I just couldn't do it. I couldn't really sit there and say, I'm withdrawing because this is too painful. I had to disappear. We went to my husband's family for Christmas, and my father-in-law looked at me and said, "You know, we would love to have more grandchildren."

Although I was feeling very low, I was determined to exhaust all my resources and not do any more drugs unless I absolutely had to. I've always been a fighter, and this was beginning to feel like a war. I started doing a lot of reading.

My husband had frequent stomachaches. He was often tired and cranky. I wondered if he had a problem with his immune system. Maybe he was missing some nutrients. I had read about Chinese medicine and acupuncture, and I thought there might be some teas he could drink that would bring him better health. I collected a number of articles for Steve to show him that this was not just some crazy idea of mine, that there were other people out there who believed in this.

I found the Pacific Institute in the phone book. We had a consultation with one of the faculty members, Dr. Z, and she said it would take four to six months to bring Steve's body into balance. She gave him a few different teas to drink. They smelled awful, but Steve is an adventurer, and when he takes something on, he is very methodical. He mixed these concoctions, put one herb in for twenty minutes and then another one for twenty more minutes, strained them, and drank them three times a day. Every week, he had to report to Dr. Z how he was feeling, his diet, his bowel movements. He got an acupuncture treatment each week. Since Dr. Z was in charge of training new doctors, there were always a lot of women and men in lab coats around him. He loved the attention, and he couldn't have been a better patient.

Six weeks later his stomachaches were gone, and he was much more relaxed and energetic. Four months after he started the work with Dr. Z, we went back to the IVF clinic to check his sperm. His sperm viability had increased considerably.

I became pregnant two months later without any intervention.

It took a year to assemble the five stories you just read. Today there is a stack of tapes on my desk, with case histo-

168 ries of people I've had the privilege to work with in my workshops and support groups. I selected two of those stories to celebrate this new edition of *Inconceivable*.

Ann, Greenwich, Connecticut ▪ *Lili, 5 lb. 8oz.*

I got married a week before my thirty-fifth birthday. A few months later, I decided to go off birth control. I was not really in a hurry to get pregnant; I'm an architect, and my career had just started taking off. Part of me was wondering what would happen to my identity if I became a mom. Almost a year went by, and I was still pretty easygoing about it. I wanted it to just be something that would happen in its own time. At the end of that year I decided to see my OB-GYN to see if anything was wrong. Looking back, I now realize that she did all the testing at the wrong time in my cycle. She also tested Eric, and we didn't get his results for six months. I kept calling and finally I got her on the phone and said: "You know, I run a service business and I want you to know you and your staff are just not cutting it." She said, "Oh, thank you so much, it's so nice to get that feedback. I'll look into it immediately." And of course, nothing changed.

At a friend's recommendation we saw Dr. S in New York. His suggestion was to go right into in-vitro fertilization. For the first cycle, they gave me the highest dose of drugs possible and I still only produced four or five eggs. Dr. S told me I was a low responder. Prior to the second cycle they put me on birth control pills in order to regulate it. They ended up canceling that cycle because I didn't have enough eggs. Later I thought that putting me on birth control the month before was not a good decision. I also felt that they didn't need to take it to the eleventh hour before canceling that cycle. It was a poorly managed process. We decided it was time to look for another clinic.

Right around that time I became part of a mind-body group, which was mostly useful because I connected with other women who were going through this. That's where I first heard about *Inconceivable*. The things Julia talked about in the book made so much sense to me. It's funny, I'm a terrible dieter, but I never saw her suggestions about food as a diet. I just thought, I have to be good to myself. And it was surprisingly easy because at that point it was so nice to have something to do that felt healthy. I started eating mostly organic vegetables and fruit, I eliminated all red meat, I started juicing. For the first time in my life I decided that I was going to get eight hours of sleep a night. So I would say: "What time is it? Okay, we're going to bed at eleven, that means I can set the clock for seven." I mean I started thinking, this is my priority, I need to take care of me. All of that was inspired by Julia's story.

In our search for a clinic we decided that the statistics didn't matter to us. We wanted a team that worked with problem cases, since clearly I was not an easy fix. At the initial consultation, Dr. G said to us that thirty-five to forty percent of his patients were women who had not been accepted into other clinics. So that spoke my language. I also had a good feeling about him as a person. He did a couple of things that I thought were smart. First, he did more hormonal testing up front in the first five days of the cycle. He said that every cycle is different and you want to make sure that before you embark on the process, you have the best cycle. He also did a number of sonograms to make sure that there weren't any eggs that were already too far along. He said, "We're just going to make sure that this is the right month, because we're not in some outrageous hurry." And then he tested very carefully when the eggs should be released. This was quite different from the clinic we had worked with previously, where they routinely treated the eggs on day eleven. Dr. G treated them on day seventeen. He just let them grow. I felt it was much more tailored to me, rather than following some arbitrary schedule. Still, I did not get pregnant that cycle, and that was hard.

One day my friend Lisa called and suggested we go to a Resolve conference. We met Julia there and picked up a flyer about her workshop. We both went into the workshop expecting basically a set of instructions: this is what you should eat, this is where you go for a colonic, etc. . . . And although there certainly was a lot of information like that, my favorite parts were the various exercises and the discussions.

Our doctor suggested that we do another IVF cycle, but after the workshop I realized I was not ready for it emotionally or spiritually. One of the things I got from Julia was the idea that I was the expert. It was something that at first didn't make a lot of sense to me, it was really very foreign to think of myself as the authority. But as I continued to work in the group I gradually began to trust myself more; to feel, yeah, with this process I am the expert. And I decided that after having put my body through all those hormones I needed a break.

I was in Julia's support group three months. The space in the group felt very safe and whole. There was a level of honesty and clearsightedness that felt so healthy to me. It was the kind of space that I wanted to be able to keep creating for myself. I also loved the movement work and the imagery exercises. I had tried visualizations before, but I was always left with this feeling that I couldn't really quiet my mind down enough to do them. This time they were very immediate; Julia would take her cues from whatever we were talking about at the moment. And when I would start to do them at home, I changed them and they became my own. The exercise that ended up being really powerful for me was being in the center of a group of women and having each of those women say something—whatever message they would want to share with me. I re-created that for myself a lot. And it changed—at some point, I saw myself walking up a mountainside and there were women along the way to help me up. And each of them had a gift for the baby, not material gifts but gifts like laughter and love. I still get chills thinking about it; these were all women that I loved and a number of them had died.

By the time the next IVF cycle came around I was in a very different place emotionally and spiritually. After the retrieval I came back to the group and said that I was disappointed, because I thought I would produce more eggs but they only retrieved two. The group's response was "You only need one, one good egg." It turned out that both eggs fertilized. They did the transfer and I was supposed to stay on the table for an hour afterward. Eric had to make a call and I found myself doing an imagery exercise. I visualized my womb as this very warm and welcoming place for the embryos, with soft lighting; the lining of the womb was a plush red sofa and my heartbeat was the music in the background. And there were these two embryos. One of them was a ten cell and one was a four cell. I had this image of these two strivers, the big, strong ten cell just swimming along, heading toward the music. And the little four cell who was like a shrimp, but it had the spirit, it was going to keep up with its sibling, trying really hard, swimming upstream. It was very real, very powerful. It was the most magical moment. I spent that weekend just lying around and resting and every once in a while I would repeat that visualization. It felt very good to do it, I didn't feel I was pushing myself in any way, it just kind of floated into my mind.

During the waiting period I was at my parents' country house, and I was convinced that it didn't work because I started getting cramps. I remember saying to Eric, "Don't get your hopes up, I feel like I'm going to get my period." There is one more important detail. In my very first IVF cycle they misread the data. They told me I was pregnant and they called me five hours later and said I wasn't. And then the third IVF, the first one at the new clinic—they told me I had a low reading. They said, "You know, it's possible that you could be pregnant, but the reading is low, we'll have to test again in a few days." It turned out the reading was something like 17. They didn't explain to me how really low that was.

So this time we did our blood test on a Friday morning and in the afternoon I called the clinic. And they said—we have a very good reading. They told me the reading was 1,039. And I couldn't understand it. I started to sob; I literally couldn't understand going from 17 to 1,039. I was sobbing and asking the nurse: "What does this number mean?" It took me a while to trust it. Everyone else around me was very optimistic, but it took a while to believe that it was real. But she is quite real, my daughter, although sometimes I still think it's all a dream.

Amy, New York, New York ■ *Eliot, 6 lb. 4 oz.*

A few months after my thirty-first birthday, I got very sick. My lymph nodes were swollen and I had constant sore throats. My body was covered with scars; my arms, legs, stomach, my chest, and my entire back were filled with them. I went to four different dermatologists and none of them could tell me what exactly was wrong with me. They took biopsies, they said it was hormonal, and they tested my follicle stimulating hormone level, which at that point came back normal.

Very slowly I began to get better, but my body changed.

174 My periods were much lighter, I started having hot flashes, and I stopped having cramps with my periods. I got very nervous and I scheduled a consultation with Dr. C, a reproductive endocrinologist at one of the New York clinics. She felt it was all in my head; she tested my FSH, which at the time was 12.5. (At the lab of this clinic anything over 10 was problematic.) I asked her if the change in my cycles signaled fertility problems. She said I just needed to calm down, and that I had nothing to worry about. This was in October. A few months later we started trying and when nothing happened for a few months I decided to see a new doctor. Luckily I brought my records along and Dr. K looked at them and said: "This is a little high, I need to test you." It turned out by then my FSH had gone up to 23.12. I remember sitting in Dr. K's office, thinking, Now I'll never get pregnant without drugs. I said to him, "If I get pregnant with twins, will that be okay since I'm so petite? Will I be able to carry them?"

He said, "I wouldn't be thinking of twins if I were you. We don't even know if you could ever get pregnant."

That's when I started to panic. And of course I left that place as fast as I could.

It took three months to see Dr. M at another clinic. He suggested we start with Clomid and after two cycles, I moved on to injectables. In June I had done my fifth cycle of the drugs and I was out of my mind, crying all the time. I used to just start crying in the middle of the afternoon at work. I would say, "Don't mind me, I'm not really upset right now, it's just this hormonal thing." So Dr. M said to me, "You are clinically depressed. Let's put you on Prozac, and let's do IVF next month."

I said, "I think I need a break."

"Taking a break would just make you more depressed," he said.

But I felt if I didn't take a break I was going to have a nervous breakdown.

Around that time my friend Lisa went to Julia's workshop and she was very excited about her approach. I don't think she had a major problem and she actually got pregnant very quickly. She said I had to read *Inconceivable*. I remember exactly where I was when I read it; it turned my head around. Suddenly I realized there could be another way out there. I was also a little intimidated and overwhelmed; wasn't sure I could do what Julia did, but there was a spark of hope.

My hot flashes were getting worse. As soon as I got off the drugs, they became quite unbearable. And my FSH was still elevated. I was going to try IVF with yet another doctor, Dr. L, but he didn't think it made sense to do it with the numbers I was getting. He was much less arrogant than any of the others. Basically he said that they didn't really know what the problem was and why I was having all those menopausal symptoms and he was very supportive of exploring any and all alternatives.

Lisa called one day and said Julia was having a workshop the following week. Something very deep and at the same time very quiet happened in that workshop for me. I realized that I could do this in my own way—that was something I held on to—the idea that each person was different and each person needed to find her own way into the work. And at the same time I came away with a lot of specific information on treatments, and food, and tools you could use to help you find out what worked best for you. The next day I started cleaning up my diet, I took a yoga class, I bought a bunch of books and started reading about herbs.

Soon after, I called Julia for a consultation, because my hot flashes were very upsetting for me. Also the night sweats were escalating. It really felt like I was going through menopause. We covered a lot in that meeting. We looked at the possible connection between the menopausal symptoms and my depressed immune system; we looked at some unresolved issues about my history, and my feelings about motherhood. Julia suggested that there was a connection between those feelings and my current difficulties. And I think I had known that for a while, but just needed someone to verbalize it for me. So after the consultation I did a lot of thinking, a lot of healing in that area. Also the whole process intensified; I started yoga classes, I completely changed my diet, which is something I never thought I could do. In the olden days, we used to have dinner parties, we used to eat out a lot—I am a gourmet chef and I used to make these elaborate meals with lots of starch, butter, sugar. We would have big desserts and wine every night. The idea of changing that seemed overwhelming. But after the workshop and the consultation there was just no stopping me. What happened was that I felt so great after just ten days of getting rid of all the junk—I had so much more energy—that I kept looking for more things to do. I felt so good that sometimes there were days when I forgot to think about the baby. Now that was huge.

At this point I was still seeing Dr. L. We were doing intra-uterine inseminations, and as before I was taking progesterone after ovulation.

I joined Julia's support group and also worked with her privately. I learned to take clues from my dreams and use imagery and work with my body in a completely new way; to listen to what was going on inside me. It was an adventure. Lots of coincidences started happening in my life. It felt like this space opened up inside me; I just knew that I was on the right track. I remember the last support group I went to; Julia talked about prayer; about praying in a more demanding way, to say exactly what we are feeling even if it's "Look, God, this is just not acceptable!" Our priest is this really funky great guy and I told him what she said and he went: Yes!!! He was all for it. I only prayed that way once, I said: "Look, God, no one is Catholic anymore, but I found a spiritual way to be Catholic, and that is how I will raise my child."

In that group we also talked about throwing away our ovulation kits for one cycle to see what it felt like. To just really take our cues from our bodies. And that's what I did. I was so focused on that kit. Throwing it out made me nervous. It was also the first month in a very long time that we didn't do intra-uterine inseminations. We just had sex. I remember going to see Dr. L two days later and he said,

"I don't know if you ovulated. You definitely didn't have enough sex this month. I want you to stop taking progesterone and see what your levels are without the drugs." But I didn't feel good about doing it. I just didn't see how he could possibly know whether we did or did not have enough sex. So not only did I stay on the progesterone, I also used the progestin on my belly.

It was Palm Sunday, the holiest time for Catholics. I went to church a lot that week and felt very moved, very connected spiritually. On Monday I found out one of my best friends was pregnant and I got pretty down about that.

Then the following week I was flossing my teeth one morning and my gums were gushing blood, which I knew is a sign of pregnancy. I went into the bedroom and said to Charles, "You know this progesterone, it tricks you. It makes you think you're pregnant when you're not." But I did a home pregnancy test and the line was so light, I didn't even tell Charles, I just ignored it. Then I decided to call the company.

I said, "Hello, I'm on progesterone, does it give you a false positive on a pregnancy test?" They said, "No."

"I have this light line . . ."

"Go to your doctor."

And I just didn't believe it the whole day. I called Charles that night and asked him to stop and pick up a pregnancy test on his way home. He said to me: "You mean an ovulation kit?"

"No, a pregnancy test."

So he picked one up, came home at nine-thirty, and I

waited till the morning to repeat the test. Again it came out very light and he wasn't excited either. Both of us were in such shock, we just couldn't quite get it. I called my doctor's office and got a lab test. The nurse left a message for me the next day and all she said was "Your HCG is 1200 but your progesterone is 13." I called her back and I said, "You mean I'm pregnant?" I was screaming and sobbing and laughing, she must've thought I'd lost it. She had progesterone delivered to my workplace and told me to take it immediately. I did oral progesterone and suppositories. It took about two weeks for the numbers to normalize. They wanted for me to really take it easy, to stay still as much as possible.

Charles and I figured out we had gone to eleven different reproductive endocrinologists in the last five years. With my numbers I allegedly had a zero to five percent chance of getting pregnant.

The baby is coming in about a week. Everything in my life changed because of all I've gone through. Everything. I am much more tuned in to my body, much nicer to myself. There is a sense of awe I feel about this new life inside me. I know I'll be a very different mother because of how I got to be one.

EPILOGUE

The experiences are similar. Somewhere along the way, each of us had to leave the certainty of our advisers behind and leap into the unknown, to follow our own wisdom which unfolded one step at a time.

At times I imagine all those longed-for babies cruising around the overworld. They're leaning over the clouds, cheering us on; waiting for the right moment to beam down. Perhaps they're just giving us a chance to re-parent ourselves first. As kindly and lovingly and generously as we hope someday to parent them.

So our best bet, I think, is to hold on to our pilgrim's stick and keep going as far as our longing takes us. One day we are bound to stand on holy ground—and for all we know someone might be there to greet us. But by then, we will have reclaimed our lives.

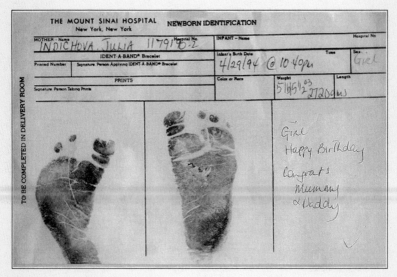

"Newborn Identification" feet.

RESOURCES

Books

The Fertile Heart Imagery Handbook: Encouraging Conception and a Healthy Birth Through Creative Visualizations. Julia Indichova. Adell Press, 2000.

Women's Bodies, Women's Wisdom: Creating Physical and Emotional Health and Healing. Christiane Northrup, M.D. Bantam Doubleday Dell Publishing Group, 1998.

The Language of Fertility: A Revolutionary Mind-Body Program for Conscious Conception. Niravi B. Payne, M.S., and Brenda Lane Richardson. Harmony Books, 1997.

Fibroid Tumors & Endometriosis. Self Help Book. Solving the problems of heavy bleeding, cramps, pain, infertility, and other symptoms associated with fibroid tumors and endometriosis. Susan M. Lark, M.D. Celestial Arts, 1993, 1995.

A Woman's Best Medicine: Health, Happiness, and Long Life Through Mahrishi Ayur-Veda. Nancy Lonsdorf, M.D., Veronica Butler, M.D., and Melanie Brown, Ph.D. G. P. Putnam's Sons, 1993.

Healing Mind, Healthy Woman: Using the Mind-Body Connection to Manage Stress and Take Control of Your Life. Alice D. Domar, Ph.D., and Henry Dreher. Henry Holt and Company, Inc., 1996.

The Woman's Encyclopedia of Natural Healing. Dr. Gary Null. Seven Stories Press, 1996.

Alternative Medicine Guide to Women's Health #1. Burton Goldberg and the editors of *Alternative Medicine.* Future Medicine Publishing, 1998.

Fertility, Cycles and Nutrition. Marilyn M. Shanon. The Couple to Couple League International Inc., 1996.

The Infertility Diet: Get Pregnant and Prevent Miscarriage. Fern Reiss. Peanut Butter and Jelly Press, 1999.

I Got Pregnant, You Can Too! How Healing Yourself Physically, Mentally and Spiritually Leads to Fertility. Katie Boland. Underwood Books, 1998.

Healing Visualizations, Creating Health Through Imagery. Gerald Epstein, M.D. Bantam Books, 1989.

You'll See It When You Believe It: The Way to Your Personal Transformation. Dr. Wayne W. Dyer. Avon Books, 1989.

Timeshifting: Creating More Time to Enjoy Your Life. Stephan Rechtshaffen, M.D. Doubleday, 1996.

You Can Heal Your Life. Louise L. Hay. Hay House, 1999.

Food and Healing: How What You Eat Determines Your Health, Your Well-being, and the Quality of Your Life. AnneMarie Colbin. Ballantine Books, 1986, 1996.

Fit for Life. Harvey and Marilyn Diamond. Warner Books, 1985.

Natural Health, Natural Medicine: A Comprehensive Manual for Wellness and Self-Care. Andrew Weil, M.D. Houghton Mifflin Company, 1995.

184 *Wise Woman Herbal for the Childbearing Years.* Susun Weed. Ash Tree Publishing, 1986.

The Couple's Guide to Fertility: Updated with the Newest Scientific Techniques to Help You Have a Baby. Gary Berger, Marc Goldstein, Mark Fuerst. Doubleday, 1995.

Dr. Richard Marrs' Fertility Book. Richard Marrs, M.D., and Lisa Friedman Bloch and Kathy Kirtland Silverman. Dell, 1997.

Preventing Miscarriage: The Good News. Jonathan Scher, M.D., and Carol Dix. HarperCollins, 1991.

Audiotapes

The Fertile Heart Imagery Tape. Julia Indichova. Produced by www.FertileHeart.com.

Holistic Fertility Treatment Options: Nutrition, Homeopathy, Herbal Medicine, Craniosacral Therapy. A panel moderated by Julia Indichova. Produced by www.FertileHeart.com, 2000.

For information about additional titles, retreats, workshops, and support groups e-mail us at info@fertileheart.com.

ACKNOWLEDGMENTS

This edition of *Inconceivable* could not have happened without the openheartedness of the women and men who read our story and used it to spark their own journeys. The two women whose stories appear in this edition have been a privilege to work with. I'm touched by the compassion that compelled them to share their experiences.

Nor could we have made it to the shores of Broadway Books without the brilliant navigation of my agent Jane Dystel, my editor Tricia Medved, and the thoughtful efforts of Miriam Goderich and James Benson. I'm grateful to each of them for their guidance and their faith in my work.

A special thank-you to Lisa Rosenthal and Carolyn Berger of the American Infertility Association, and Maris Meyerson and Jane T. of Resolve of Northern California, who gave me a thumbs-up when I most needed it.

My appreciation for the help I received with writing the book has only deepened over the last several years. So, here once again, I wish to acknowledge my original encouragers.

186   The five sister warriors who entrusted me with the stories for the first edition made an enormous contribution to this project.

Robert Wolf, Roger Frank, Linda Harms, Dorothy Crystal Ross, Betsy Agoglia, and John Beaulieu ran alongside me for the length of the race. My deepest gratitude and love to each.

Many friends listened, read, and contributed valuable ideas. A huge thank-you to Anne Tobias, Lois Nachamie, Sallie Sanborn, Carol Clements, Amy Mereson, Sandra Marcus, Vivi Mansukhani, Lisa Marfleet, Ellen Carter, Sparrow, Royce Froelich, Rikki Asher, Merrill Goldstein, Ted Shapiro, Janet Grillo, Lynn Giudici, Linda Beller, and Jeff Langer.

My father, Oskar Indich, my sister, Susan, her husband, Richard Diamond, and my nephews Alexis, Matthew, and Steven have been my staunch supporters.

My aunt Lillian Lenovits was my most patient first English teacher and editor.

Lillian and Miles Cahn, my guardian angels of the last twenty-eight years, devised the title and cheered me on.

Sandra Dorr and Susan Shapiro, the world's greatest editors, have been a joy to work with. Their guidance was invaluable in bringing the manuscript to its final form.

I would have been unable to write a single word without Elizabeth Bieganska and the wonderful staff of the Morningside Montessori School, who kept my children happy and safe.

Never, ever, has anyone been on my side as unconditionally as my first editor, book designer, graphic artist, photographer, guru, chef, and the most amazing father and husband, Edward Nathan Baum. My three miracles, Ed, Ellena, and Adi, have given me a life that in my wildest dreams I could not have imagined.

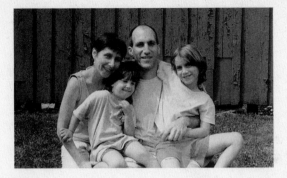

ABOUT THE AUTHOR

Julia Indichova has been researching holistic approaches to fertility since her own diagnosis in 1992. Her work has been published in the *New York Times,* the *San Francisco Chronicle, Healthy and Natural,* and a number of other publications. She is the founder of the webzine FertileHeart.com and the director of the Fertile Heart Learning Center in Woodstock, New York. Julia runs ongoing support groups and workshops in New York City and Woodstock, and travels around the country speaking about fertility, women's issues, and health empowerment.

Visit Julia's website at www.fertileheart.com